BLOOD, BREAD, AND ROSES

BLOOD, BREAD, AND ROSES

How Menstruation Created the World

• • •

JUDY GRAHN

BEACON PRESS . BOSTON

Beacon Press
25 Beacon Street
Boston, Massachusetts 02108-2892

Beacon Press Books
are published under the auspices of
the Unitarian Universalist Association of Congregations.

99 98 97 96 95 94 93   8 7 6 5 4 3 2 1

Text design by Gwen Frankfeldt

Library of Congress Cataloging-in-Publication Data

Grahn, Judy, 1940–
Blood, bread, and roses: how menstruation created the world / Judy Grahn.
p.   cm.
Includes bibliographical references and index.
ISBN 0-8070-7504-3
1. Menstruation—Social aspects.   2. Menstruation—Cross-cultural studies.
I.Title.
GN484.38.G73   1993
392′.14—dc20   93-7701

To poets

Contents

Foreword

M O D E R N culture positions itself in opposition to nature. Western culture—at least since the Pythagorean table of opposites was formalized in the sixth century B.C.E.—associates the male with admirable normative principles and the female with the vague and indeterminate, the unbounded and formless, the irregular and disorderly. Patriarchal culture demeans and denies the elemental power of the female body. Not surprisingly, then, modern Western patriarchal culture renders the moon tides of women's bodies, the very blood that feeds the continuation of the human species, invisible and irrelevant if properly hidden, or shameful and unclean if not. This response is generally considered natural and inevitable.

Judy Grahn's *Blood, Bread, and Roses* turns that vast cultural construction inside out. Her boldly original interpretation of cultural history challenges the assumption that because menstruation is largely hidden and inconsequential in modern society it must, therefore, have always been so. Across the great divide from such embarrassingly messy and *uncontrollable* seepage as menstrual blood, it is understood, the triumphal march of progress—conceptual thought, language, mathematics, and technology—gradually led humans from primate consciousness to the fully evolved status of *Homo faber, Homo oeconomicus, Homo aestheticus.* Grahn demonstrates, however, that if one refuses to ignore the elemental presence and processes of the female body, the cultural history of our species looks quite different.

In *Blood, Bread, and Roses* Grahn focuses on the meanings of *separation* in cross-cultural responses to menstruation. She first considers the origin myths of many cultures and notes that a high proportion of them begin with an undifferentiated space/time, an era of chaos and indeterminate form, from which creation occurs via separation: the separation of land from water, of earth from sky, of rivers from oceans, of mountains from plains. Grahn speculates that the foundation of so many origin stories—a time of undifferentiation—may be an extremely resilient reference to early humans' "crossing of the great abyss" from primate consciousness to the eventual development of conceptualizing, abstracting human consciousness. For this to occur, consciousness had to become externalized, that is, linked with events outside the human in ways that led to apprehension of patterns and concepts. Grahn believes that this pivotal development must have occurred in relation to females' dawning awareness that their 29.5-day menstrual cycle of bleeding was in rhythm with—and hence related to—an external object, the white moon in the sky. The resultant consciousness, which she calls "the menstrual mind," became externalized and displayed, particularly because of the necessity for females to teach their discovery to members of the group who did not menstruate. Males learned the *metaforms,* Grahn's term for various expressions of menstrual logic, such as principles of separation, synchronic relationship, and cyclical time. Eventually the males extended the metaforms, rearranged them, and mirrored them back to the females, creating what Grahn sees as "an ongoing dance of mind between the genders."

Grahn then considers ways in which the central concept of separation has been expressed in a wide variety of menstrual seclusion rituals. The three most common aspects of *taboo* (a Polynesian word for menstruation) for a secluded menstruant were that she must be strictly separated from water, light, and the earth; she was also prohibited from being touched and from touching her own

body. If she were to go to the river, for instance, and drink a hand-
ful of water, her own moon-blood waters might well mix with the
other waters, causing all separation to unravel, plunging the world
back into the undifferentiated, chaotic state. Cross-culturally, eth-
nographers of native cultures have often been told that women's
rites hold the world in balance.

Other cultural historians have noted that the Upper Paleolithic
bone calendars (bones with notches in groups of numbers that
usually add up to 29.5 or 30) establish the link between lunar/
menstrual observations and counting. Hence from the menstrual
mind came the beginnings of measurement, arithmetic, geometry,
and all mathematics. Grahn, however, goes much further, tracing
the results of menstrual logic as its practices and paraphernalia migrated from the site of menstrual seclusion (usually a menstrual
hut) into society.

Since the menstruant was to mark the end of her dark-of-the-
moon days by emerging at dawn into the light, the door of the
menstrual hut faced east, an orientation that was replicated in ceremonial buildings and dwellings and has been maintained for millennia in diverse native cultures. Since the menstruant's successful
observation of the separation rites carried cosmological significance, her emergence was met with celebration and feasting, for
which ceremonial food, elaborate dress, and bodily decoration
were devised. (Until recent times, women probably had compara-
tively few menstrual cycles in their lifetime because of frequent
pregnancies and extended periods of lactation.) The most elaborate
celebration followed the longest and most exacting menstrual seclusion, that of menarche, a woman's first menstrual period.

In a fascinating discussion of "parallel menstruations," Grahn
cites a variety of rituals that replicate the disciplines of menstrual
seclusion. (She notes that a central meaning of the Sanskrit word
for ritual, *r'tu,* is menstruation, the original ritual.) In many cultures hunting, which appeared in human history much later than
menses, borrowed menstrual-like rites of seclusion and privation
for hunters prior to an excursion. Much later, when rituals to bene-

fit the entire society were performed by special groups who became the priestly caste, the aristocracy, and royalty, many concepts issuing from menstrual logic were again adopted.

Grahn also demonstrates the effect of menstrual logic in symbolization, narrative, and the evolution of godheads, as well as in the development of art, handicraft, and technology. In time, production and technological endeavors took on a life of their own, ushering in the age of materialism and a corresponding diminution of rituals of cosmological reciprocity. With that transformation our species crossed another abyss, Grahn feels, this time to the "logic of male blood power," including ritualized warfare. She ends by suggesting ways in which we might unravel the contemporary "necroforms" of exploitation and destruction to achieve political and cultural renewal.

What is one to make of this grand theory? First, it is important to keep in mind that Grahn states that she is presenting a female-centered origin story. It is intended, I believe, to take a long-overdue place on the table for discussion alongside the towering stack of androcentric theories and assumptions about cultural history. With regard to the possible objection that Grahn's thesis is reductionist, one should bear in mind that she never denies dynamics other than the one that is her focus, that she is a poet who theorizes with a brilliantly associative mind, and that the lost history of menstrual logic must be writ large in order to get onto the discussion table in modern times at all. In response to the possible objection that "all this" is nothing new since reproduction has long been understood as important in the early shaping of cultural history, Grahn emphasizes her finding that it was women's moon-blood, not babies, that was considered numinous. (If so, this realization might explain the absence of infants from the upper paleolithic and neolithic goddess statues.) Other feminist authors have speculated on the early significance *for women* of women's blood mysteries, but Grahn traces their effect on culture, invention, production, trade, science, religion, and more.

The appearance of *Blood, Bread, and Roses* is particularly

timely in relation to at least three fields of knowledge: feminist theory, linguistics, and social constructivism (also called "social constructionism" or "deconstructive postmodernism"). Feminist theory is a wide-ranging, interdisciplinary endeavor to analyze critically the patriarchal bias in scholarship and to broaden the range of perception, insight, logic, concern, and activist implications. Grahn's thesis on the centrality of cultural responses to menses is surely relevant to the current multiperspectival efforts in history, anthropology, psychology, and other fields, in which a plurality of interpretations is valued. Moreover, this book joins works of body-oriented feminist cultural theory that include, for example, *Of Woman Born* by Adrienne Rich, *Woman and Nature* by Susan Griffin, *The Politics of Reproduction* by Mary O'Brien, and *The Politics of Women's Spirituality* by myself and others.

Regarding linguistic theory, Grahn seems to have independently arrived—via her poetic mind—at a realization about conceptual thinking that has recently rumbled through that field. Prior to the late 1970s, metaphor was considered a poetic device, an artifice quite distinct from objective thought and expression. It is now recognized, however, that nearly all abstract thought in humans is organized metaphorically (see, for example, *Metaphors We Live By* by George Lakoff and Mark Johnson). In addition, bodily experience has been recognized recently as being enormously influential in the evolution of metaphorical concepts (see *The Body in the Mind* by Mark Johnson). Grahn's thesis suggests rich possibilities in both of these areas, for she not only proposes the metaphors of menstrual logic but also introduces the concept of "metaforms," cultural practices or objects that embody those metaphors.

With regard to the grip of social constructivism (or deconstructionism) on much academic and other intellectual activity these days, the accumulation of cross-cultural evidence cited in Grahn's work argues against the constructivist belief that concepts about gender and the body (or anything else) are merely "arbitrary social constructions." Deconstructionists assert that one can know nothing about the body or bodily experience since all one really knows are the received concepts about such matters in one's particular society. Contrary to the claims of this belief system, culture *responds to* the elemental power of the female body, not the other way around. By that I mean that the cultural response may be positive or negative but it is extremely unlikely that any early society *did not notice* the moon rhythms of the female and her procreative capabilities. A number of recently published feminist books have critiqued the disembodied orientation of deconstructive postmodernism, such as *Nothing Mat(t)ers* by Somer Brodribb, *Unbearable Weight* by Susan Bordo, and my own *States of Grace*. Grahn's *Blood, Bread, and Roses* contributes to the efforts to examine the social and historical construction of concepts in ways that acknowledge our embodiment and our embeddedness in subtle processes of earth community and the cosmos. Theorists in this cluster call such an alternative "*embodied* postmodernism" or "*ecological* postmodernism."

Finally, I would like to share a general sense of my personal responses to reading this book. In 1979 I commissioned an article from Judy Grahn on menstruation for my anthology, *The Politics of Women's Spirituality*. I supplied the title, "From Sacred Blood to the Curse and Beyond"; she supplied an extraordinary article—which, by the way, led the women of the editorial department at Beacon Press to commission this book and to wait patiently through many years of research. I wanted women to be able to get beyond "the curse," the culturally implanted embarrassment, alienation, and, for some, even self-loathing that accompanies menstruation in our society. I was aware of gloriously celebratory menarche rituals in various native cultures, yet the chasm between those orientations and that of my own culture seemed so vast as to devour efforts at imagining a different way of being. Even the subversively joyful menarche rituals some of us have created for our daughters seem dwarfed by the negative cultural messages they receive outside of our circles.

In *Blood, Bread, and Roses* the comprehensive nature of Grahn's vision gradually creates a world in which the female reader feels at home, perhaps for the first time, because Grahn brings women from the margins of cultural history to the center—as *embodied* women. Yet the author also incorporates an all-too-familiar story of a contemporary woman's struggle—her own—to escape the abhorrence with which she viewed her menses. The contrast in this book between the rich tapestry of women's lost history and the modern, barren version of the female's cultural significance that shaped the lives of the author and her mother creates a poignant declaration of the need to recover the embodied wisdom that once was ours.

It feels to me as if this book is a huge bouquet of red roses offered lovingly to women everywhere, a gift that gives us back our history, our presence, and our existential grounding. It frees women from feeling like trespassers when we venture outside of domestic space into the realms of the arts, science, trade, education, and religion— for the wellsprings of human culture may well have flowed red. Whatever the extent of the importance of menstrual logic in various societies, *Blood, Bread, and Roses* stands against its eradication from cultural history any longer.

As I was reading the manuscript, I often exclaimed to my husband, "Amazing! Listen to this!" After several days of this unsolicited crash course in the Grahnian perspective, he remarked wryly, "It seems unfair that men don't get to menstruate. Fortunately, though, some of us get to *live with* people who do."

Exactly so.

Charlene Spretnak

All Blood Is Menstrual Blood

I M A G E S of blood are all around us, everywhere in our modern, urbanized society blood is depicted, spoken of, displayed: the blood of wound, of death and to a lesser extent birth is part of daily viewing in television and films; we are completely familiar with the bloodlines of kinship, and with the blood of violence, of murder and vengeance, of sacrifice, suffering, and of IV drug users; the blood of warning, of wounding, of threat; the danger attached to the blood of AIDS; the blood of life, of transfusions, and of redemption; the blood of Christ; the blood of martyrdom, of St. Sebastian, of the prize fighter depicted in the movies. Blood is genealogy in bloodlines, family blood, the blood that is thicker than water. Blood is in name and in common expression, in the blood of the lamb, in the blood of blood, sweat, and tears, in the blood of the Sangre de Christo Mountains, in the blood of blood brothers, the blood of the stigmata, the blood on the moon, the blood that cannot be squeezed from turnips, the blood dripping from the mouth of the vampire, the bloodstain on Lady Macbeth's hands, the blood gurgling down the shower drain in horror films. Real blood is everywhere in our society, Saturday-night blood, drive-by-shooting blood, the blood he was covered in after he was shot, or stabbed, or blown up; the pencil thin line like a necklace across her throat, the great spread of it when she was chopped up, the bloody nose, the bleeding ulcer, the sting of hemmorrhoids, the blood on the surgeon's gown and the butcher's apron, the many rivers of battle and massacre that have run with blood, the battlefield soaked, the sand reddened, the blood on the child's ear and the wife's mouth and the young man's cheek. In the cities the gutters are streaming and sidewalks pooled and car seats puddled and emergency rooms smeared and police clubs stained. When gangster John Dillinger's body fell on the street, shot by the FBI and spouting from numerous holes, passersby instantly leaped as though to a holy stream, to dip a handkerchief, newspaper, even a sleeve, into the blood of his wounds, to take a bit home with them. Blood is magic, blood is holy, and wholly riveting of our attention.

Menstrual blood is the only source of blood that is not traumatically induced. Yet in modern society, this is the most hidden blood, the one so rarely spoken of and almost never seen, except privately by women, who shut themselves in a little room to quickly and in many cases disgustedly change their pads and tampons, wrapping the bloodied cotton so it won't be seen by others, wrinkling their faces at the odor, flushing or hiding the evidence away. Blood is everywhere, and yet the one, the only, the single name it has not publicly had for many centuries, is menstrual blood. Menstrual blood, like water, just flows. Its fountain existed long before knives or flint; menstruation is the original source of blood.

Menstrual is blood's secret name. All blood is menstrual blood.

A Woman's First Bleeding: My Menarche

In a few months I will turn thirteen; the event I have prayed for more than a year never to happen to me will happen to me. God will not intervene to turn me into a boy at the last minute. I will be near tears as my mother fumbles her explanation and display of how to wear a sanitary pad. I cannot tell whether her troubled expression is from embarrassment, sorrow, or fear that my life will now resemble hers.

"Why, why," I wail suddenly. "Boys don't bleed, why do I have to, it isn't fair!"

"So you can have babies; it happens to all women," she replies. But I know this is inaccurate, for I know that our spinster neighbors have no babies. I have discussed this at length with God, angling for a bargain. "I don't want babies, so menstruation is wasted on me," is my most excellent argument. Anyhow, why does it have to happen so many times, why not once for each baby? My outrage and disillusion burst out in whining, furious tones. "Why doesn't this happen to boys, and why"—I look at the betraying red stuff on my fingertips—"why is God so <u>mean</u> to girls?"

My mother answers with resigned logic, "Boys have to shave, boys have to go to war. It all evens out." From the age of eleven, I prayed to be turned into a boy not only to avoid menstruation but out of dread for all the apparent female biological dictates: breasts, babies, marriage. I also avoided all manner of "girl things," including jump rope, jacks and hopscotch. I associated them with restriction, declining mind, lack of expression and power in the world, and general silliness. Not for me the secrets girls began telling each other, the all-night slumber parties where, I now discover, they did amazing things, like "levitating" each other to the ceiling.

While other girls played girl games, I identified with my father's presents, a rubber snake and a hairy spider on a string, and cap guns with holsters. When I turn twelve he gives me a 22-caliber rifle and takes me shooting. "So you can protect yourself," he explains, "and if you ever get too poor to buy food you can always take this out to the woods and shoot something to eat." A practical Swedish-born man, raised in the rural area of Illinois of the early twentieth century, when squirrel-and-rabbit stew was regular fare.

I love all his presents, though my mother does not; the more gunlike they are, the more she hates them. But I have already decided that I don't want to be like her, so I don't care. The girls at school go through their adolescent changes together. They stop displaying either their intelligence or physical prowess; they apply cosmetics and new ways of walking; they talk of nothing but boys, to whom they are alternatingly obsequious and manipulative; they diet continually, examining each other ounce by ounce, and they become a complete mystery to me. I continue as though a boy, hoping this will please the universe enough for it to give me an ungirl niche in which to live.

A few weeks after my first blood, my father brings what from the joy on his face I know he considers the most wonderful present of all. My parents sit silent in one unit as, surprised and eager, I unwrap it. What special mysterious objects could this handsome, weighty case contain? Will I open to a row of silvery exacto knives with special blades and drills for woodworking, or a longed-for chemistry set, or—dared I hope—a box of engineer's tools, some calipers, a plumb bob, even a slide rule? My eager fingers slacken and nearly let the case fall as the mirror on the inside flap comes into view, and then the shining row of tubes, the soft dark brushes, the little rounds of colors, the heavier round jar marked "rouge." I am deeply humiliated.

"Oh," I say in falling tones, "oh, it's a box of cosmetics," and to my father's (and my own) hurt bafflement, I reject it.

Even while treasuring their cosmetic cases, other girls my age and from similar backgrounds went through menarchal experiences of shame and silence. Their mothers, like mine, said little or nothing to them about their menarchal passage, but for a Wintu girl of the California coastal tribes of the nineteenth century, menarche was the occasion for intense attention from her family and also from her village:

At the time of puberty, a girl notified her mother or grandmother, who then built a small brush shelter some 20 or 30 yards from the family dwelling. The girl stayed in seclusion for one to several months. The girl was not permitted to cook for herself; her diet was limited to acorn soup, prepared by the mother or grandmother. She was not supposed to leave her hut except at night. If she had to go out in the day, she covered her head with a basket or a hide. Sleep during the first five days of the first menses was forbidden, since dreams at this time were considered prejudicial to health and sanity. The girl was not to touch herself and so a head scratcher was used; this could be any twig at hand. Combing her hair was forbidden. Her cheeks were streaked with vertical lines of charcoal or red and blue pigment. During the seclusion, the elderly people gave the girl advice and instruction on her future behavior. During the period of isolation young people might sing and dance outside the adolescent's lodge at night; many of the songs were [sexual]. [In the fall a special dance to honor several girls brought groups from neighboring villages, who arrived singing and with gifts of food. The festivities lasted at least five days.] Poorer girls wore new maple-bark skirts; richer ones were dressed in buckskin aprons and were laden with beads or seeds. They carried deerhoof rattles and spirally striped ceremonial staffs. (Heizer, *Handbook of North American Indians*, vol. 8, p. 328)

During the nineteenth century and into the early twentieth, Western observers gathered hundreds of reports of attitudes toward menstruation from around the world. Many nineteenth-century peoples regarded menstrual blood with extreme respect, even fear, constructing taboos to protect themselves from impurity, illness, or death. Reports from our own day range from people who show little concern about the flow (in New Guinea, a woman may sit on the porch with a little moss under her, but otherwise her period isn't noticed), to those who stage an elaborate menarchal rite as an event of crucial social importance to everyone (for example, the beautiful Kinaaldá ceremony of the Navajo), to tampax-wearing Western women, for whom menstruation is no more than a biological given.

Perhaps the grandmother of the Wintu girl in early California might have told her an origin story that centered in menstruation, but no one in my family had stories for me. Such stories, if they existed, were lost centuries ago. My mother could barely say words pertaining to menstruation; she spoke them in a whisper, making certain no one else was nearby. In any case, at the time of my menarche, my parents and I were an isolated unit with none of our family near. No grandmother, no aunts, no community of women existed to give me menstrual instruction, seclusion, or to lead me into a public dance. Not that I missed this, at the time. I wanted simply to forget my new menstrual status, to get out into the exciting world to make my mark.

From 1971 through 1976 I lived in an all-women's household. In the context of five years in this secular women's cloister, I discovered a terrible gap in myself and in the world, the missing Greater Feminine, missing in public life, and missing in the origin stories of history, science, art, religion, and literature.

I immersed myself in the perspectives of writers who had found remnants of the "Female Principle" in the poetry of myth and the graphics of archaeology: Elizabeth Gould Davis, Evelyn Reed, Esther Harding, Jane Ellen Harrison, H.D., Gertrude Stein, Adrienne Rich, Audre Lorde, and men like Robert Graves, Frederick Engels, Robert Briffault, James Mellaart, and Eric Neumann. I was impressed also by the courage of Anton Chiekh Diop, who spent years insisting that classical Egypt had black African origins, not the European roots stated in history texts. I thought that the contributions of women to culture could have been coopted in a similar manner.

In 1973, I embarked on my own investigation and was immediately drawn to menstruation because of its connection to the lunar cycle and to time, and because the iconography of ancient temples revealed a powerful, indisputable feminine presence. Time and orientation, I learned from Gerald S. Hawkins's measurements of Stonehenge and other ancient sites, was kept in temples; and I realized menstruation, with its connection to time, could have given us early sciences. As I researched, I wrote books that, like Hansel and Gretel's bread crumbs, lead to this one. In 1972, I wrote a set of female-centered poems, *She Who;* in 1980, an article crediting menstruation with sciences of measurement, "From Sacred Blood to the Curse and Beyond"; in 1982, a myth of Helen of Troy as a "stolen" goddess, *The Queen of Wands;* in 1986, a lesbian version of the ancient Sumerian Descent myth of Inanna, *The Queen of Swords;* and in 1988, I completed a novel that ends with a menarchal rite, *Mundane's World.*

By 1983 I had also turned what was originally one chapter intended for this book into a Gay and Lesbian cultural history, *Another Mother Tongue: Gay Words, Gay Worlds*. With that work, I came to understand that origin stories are incomplete (and inaccurate) unless both genders are included, and unless many different cultures are taken into account.

Over the years, in addition to reading ethnography and mythology, I talked to many women about menstruation, participated in modern versions of menstrual rite, and saw how women reacted warmly to receiving red flowers during their periods, at weekly "Gatherings" held for two years in Oakland, California, by Paula Gunn Allen, with my assistance.

During the intensive last two and a half years of writing, I stayed in virtual seclusion, wore my hair long for "flow," ate mostly red foods, drank red beer, and wore a vest of French silk with a layered pattern of red, black, purple, and gold flowers, designed by the artist Rose Frances and sewed by her and other women I love. I thought the spirits of all our ancestors gathered around to cheer me on.

Acknowledgments

I AM grateful for financial, spiritual, and daily mental support from Kris Brandenburger, and weekly understanding and enthusiasm from Betty DeShong Meador, the two best friends a book ever had; and for library assistance and comments from Karen Sjöholm, Cosi Fabian, Rose Frances, Melvin Kettner, Jack Foley, Dawn McGuire, Lisa Carruthers, Ruth Rhoten, Alicia Ostriker, and others. Thanks to Leonard and Joyce Brandenburger for their support. Special gratitude to Charlene Spretnak, who in 1980 commissioned the original article, "From Sacred Blood to the Curse and Beyond," from what was then a complex outline called *Blood and Bread and Roses*, publishing it in her anthology, *The Politics of Women's Spirituality*. I want to thank all the kind people who gave me information, articles, books, and encouragement, among whom are Emily Culpepper, Willyce Kim, Savina J. Teubal, Katharyn Aal, Mary Beth Edelson, Kate Rosenblatt, Robin Song, Susan Thompson, Janet Capone, Harriet Ziskin, Robert Glück, Anne Cameron, Coletta Reid, Casey Czarnik, Paula Gunn Allen, the late June Arnold, the late Audre Lorde, and the late Anne Shellabarger. For early support with the project in the 1970s, I want to thank the women of Diana Press and of Mama Bears Coffeehouse in Oakland. Finally, special thanks to my excellent and gentle editor, Lauren Bryant, and to Beacon Press for their patience over the past twelve years, especially Wendy Strothman, Marie Cantlon, and Joanne Wyckoff.

I also want to acknowledge other works on theories of menstruation and culture: *The Wise Wound* by Penelope Shuttle and Peter Redgrove, *Blood Relations* by Chris Knight, *Menstruation and Menopause* by Paula Weideger, and Barbara Walker's entry "Menstruation," in *The Woman's Encyclopedia of Myths and Secrets*.

Part One

. . . B L O O D . . .
Wilderness Metaform

Chapter 1

■■■■■■■■■■■■■■■■■■■■■■■

How Menstruation Created
the World

T H E menstrual rites reported in the nineteenth century often seem cruel to us: girls had to sit in one position for days, even weeks; they ate in a strange manner, and sometimes they were tied up and "smoked" in hammocks or underwent other ordeals. Some of the chroniclers of these practices, including James Frazer, who collected voluminous material for *The Golden Bough*, were horrified at what they saw as gross mistreatment of young women; they saw the rites as a form of punishment. Yet these elaborate, strict, and bizarre-seeming rites are full of information about how menstruation has formed human character, shaped who we are, how we behave toward each other, how we hold our bodies as we walk about on the earth, and how we came to use the idea and word "earth."

I, too, was initially horrified at the extremity of some of the accounts, and at first I imagined that men had imposed a brutal system on helpless young women. But writing in 1927, in *The Mothers,* Robert Briffault had a different interpretation: "The terms in which many of our accounts are couched are calculated to suggest that those observances are imposed upon the women by the brutal tyranny and ignorant superstition of the men but . . . the women, in carrying out their arduous duties, never do so under compulsion, even where the men are most tyrannical . . . women, it appears from most accounts, segregate themselves of their own accord; they isolate themselves without consulting the men; they warn the latter not to approach them."[1]

Later, as anthropologists learned tribal languages and asked more penetrating questions, and as the twentieth-century feminist movement encouraged women to speak and write themselves, other stories emerged, suggesting that some women saw menstrual seclusion as a welcome rest from chores and a pleasant way to spend time with female companions, to drink tea together and talk. Anthropologists like Jane C. Goodale and Margaret Mead reported detailed menarchal ceremonies that were connected to weddings and to training young women in sacred lore, weaving, cooking, and caring for their families and communities.[2]

During the 1970s I struggled to find what contributions women had made to the development of science and culture. I realized that the wealth of material on taboo gathered by James Frazer and Robert Briffault made a completely new kind of sense if I looked at the female origins of the power of blood. I had begun my theorizing in the early 1970s with the argument that menstruation—because of its relation to the moon—was the most likely earliest source of the sciences of geometry, mathematics, and formal measurement.[3] Later, as I considered menstrual seclusion rites and other menstrual practices in terms of origin stories, I began to see that menstruation was a possible source, not only for science, but for everything that makes us human. I began to wonder what the contradictory information about seclusion rites and other menstrual practices might look like if we considered that women, not men, established them? I took the perspective that people institute rites for rational, not irrational, purposes, and that in all probability each gender created its own rites. It followed that *women's* logic must lie at the base of menstrual rituals.

As a poet, I understand myth as a form of factual story—provided we comprehend something of its context, its probable intent, and perhaps what its tellers consider "true." Social myths can deeply affect the viewpoint of both history and anthropology. In this examination of cultural roots, I treat myths, anthropological reports, personal memories and observations, historic accounts, and creation stories as equally valid sources of information from which to construct a pan-human mythology, a menstrual origin story. Conscientious tracing of sources is one of the cornerstones both of good science and of good mythology, and I have been careful to retain sources so accounts can be checked in their original contexts.

One word recurs again and again in stories of menstrual ritual: taboo. The word comes from Polynesian *tapua*, meaning both "sacred" and "menstruation," in the sense, as some traditions say, of "the woman's friend."[4] Besides sacred, taboo also means forbidden, valuable, wonderful, magic, terrible, frightening, and immutable law. Taboo is the emphatic use of imperatives, yes or no, you must or you must not. Taboo draws attention, strong attention, and is in and of itself a language for ideas and customs.

The taboos surrounding menstruation were restrictive laws carried out sometimes to the point of death. The exacting demands reveal the deep power with which believers endowed menstruation, with its close connections to life and death. Western reports say that tribal men were sometimes so frightened of female blood as to believe that a single drop could kill them, that even the gaze of a menstruating woman could mean death, that if her hands touched their weapons they would come to great harm on the hunt. But it is not only in the nineteenth-century accounts of tribal peoples that we find menstruation hedged with rules. The word "regulation" is linked to menstruation in European languages in the same way "taboo" is in Polynesian (though without also meaning "sacred"). In German, menstruation is *Regel,* in French *regle,* and in Spanish *las reglas.* All these words mean "measure" or "rule" as well as "menstruation" and are cognate with the terms regulate, regal, regalia, and *rex* (king). In Latin, *regula* means "rule." These terms thus connect menstruation to orderliness, ceremony, law, leadership, royalty, and measurement.

Ritual, from Sanskrit *r'tu,* is any act of magic toward a purpose. *Rita,* means a proper course. *Ri,* meaning birth, is the root of red,

5

pronounced "reed" in Old English and still in some modern English accents (New Zealand). *R'tu* means menstrual, suggesting that ritual began as menstrual acts. The root of *r'tu* is in "arithmetic" and "rhythm"; I hear it also in "art," "theater," and perhaps in "root" as well. The Sanskrit term is still alive in India, where goddess worship continues to keep *r'tu* alive in its menstrual senses; *r'tu* also refers to special acts of heterosexual intercourse immediately following menstruation, and also to specific times of year.[5]

While in Latin *menses,* meaning "month," means the menstrual flow, in Scottish *mense* meant "propriety, grace." The family of words that revolves around the English word "menstruation" includes mental, memory, meditation, mensurate, commensurate, meter, mother, mana, magnetic, mead, maniac, man, and menstruation's twin, moon.

Of old, before people thought of human generation in terms of seed and egg, many cultures believed the fetus was formed in the womb by the clotting of menstrual blood. For a multitude of peoples, menstrual blood was the primary life force, the generative principle. In birth rites, which are often similar to menstrual rites, it is the blood that is central to the restrictions; birth rites too are blood rites. Clearly menstruation is related to beginnings, and in trying to see how it is related to our cultural as well as our biological beginnings, I began to think of what differentiates us from animals. Differences that seem fundamental are two: the way we menstruate and that we externalize our ideas in language and significant material decoration and objects—in our external culture.

Our simian relatives menstruate; other animals show a bit of blood as part of their ovulatory cycle, too. Like our distant cousin apes, we are in and out of "heat," or estrus, throughout the year, rather than undergoing one period of rut in the fall as the bear and deer do, or two or three periods of estrus as mice, dogs, and cats do. Sexual connection is thus constant and keeps our species in face-to-face tension all year round.

According to anthropologist Chris Knight, the menstrual cycle of primates varies greatly, some species having a seven-day cycle, while others go all the way to thirty-nine days. Only the rhesus macaque, at a twenty-nine-day cycle, is close to the human pattern. Only the human cycle, at twenty-nine and a half days, coincides with the cycle of the moon.[6]

Unlike the estrus of any other primates, then, human menstruation is linked to a single, large, visible, external body. The onset of human menstruation can be measured by a cycle outside itself, and once that connection was realized, it was used to articulate other connections. Humans have a fundamental and unique tool of external-internal measurement in the synchronization of the menstrual cycle and the lunar cycle.

In considering menstruation as female power, in contemplating creation stories and the uniqueness of the human capacity for elaborating culture, I fashioned a new myth of origin, based at once in the body, the mind, and the spirit.

Creation Stories

Origin stories remember a time before anything was, a time that consisted entirely of darkness, of water, of endless space, or of flatness without landscape; a time before name, before consciousness; a time described as asleep, or dreaming, or by the Greek word *chaos,* meaning "yawning."

For the Tsimshian Indians of North America, as for many peoples, in the beginning "the whole world was covered with darkness."[7] For the Hopi people of the American Southwest, in the beginning of the First World was Tokpela, "Endless Space." "But first, they say, there was only the Creator, Taiowa. All else was endless space. There was no beginning and no end, no time, no shape, no life. Just an immeasurable void that had its beginning and end, time, shape, and life in the mind of Taiowa the Creator."[8]

For the ancient Greeks, creation began with the separation of

7

Earth and Sky. This version of the Greek creation myth, from Euripides, is specified as having been handed down from the female lineage:

> this is not my story
> but one my mother tells
>
> once Sky and Earth were one
> then they split in   two
>
> father and mother of all
>
> brought into light
> trees
> birds
> beasts
> fish in the sea
> race of living men[9]

According to Hesiod, "First of all there came Chaos, /and after him came/Gaia of the broad breast . . ."[10]

Creation was a matter of awakening for peoples of Australia: "The aborigines believe that, even before there was any life, the earth had always existed as a flat, featureless plain, extending on all sides to the edge of the universe. At some ill-defined period, poetically known as the 'Dream-time,' giant semi-human beings, resembling animals in their appearance but acting like men and women, rose miraculously out of the level plains under which they had been slumbering for countless ages. As these mythical beings wandered over the countryside, they created the topography: the sea coasts, the swamp-lands, the rivers and the mountain ranges."[11]

In the ancient Babylonian account of creation, nothing could be until it had a name; once named, it existed:

> Long since, when above the heaven had not been named,
> when the earth beneath (still) bore no name,
> when the ocean (*apsu*), the primeval, the generator of them, and
> the originator (?) Tiamat, who brought forth them both—
> their waters were mingled together.[12]

In this version, dated by scholarly agreement to the early part of the second millennium B.C.E.; though the story itself must reach back much further, to a beginning of human consciousness, heaven and earth are imagined as "waters" mingling in an undifferentiated state. The images of heaven and earth, of the originator goddess, Tiamat, and of Apsu (*apsu*), her male mate, constantly overlap. Tiamat mingles her waters with the primal ocean. She herself has been identified as the ocean, as "bitter waters," that is, salty waters, menstrual fluids. Apsu, the Abyss, is the "sweet waters," that is, semen. Tiamat has also been called "the Great Watery Abyss."[13]

As "bitter waters," Tiamat describes the salty nature of menstrual blood carried to its greatest earthly denominator, the sea. She is the Red Sea; the Arab name for the eastern shore of the Red Sea is *Tihamat*. She has been called "Ocean of Blood." Tiamat is menstruation externalized, a complex metaphor about the nature of the earth and other elements. In Egypt, she was Temu or Te-Mut, oldest of deities. In Greek, her name is "Goddess Mother," in Latin *dia mater*. She is measurement/mother/originator by means of *dia*, two; that is to say, she is creation through separation. Her name is Diameter, horizon, the line that separates heaven and earth, sky and ocean.[14]

The idea of Tiamat as original water occurs in the creation story in Genesis, chapter 1, as *tehom*, "the deep." This creation story is believed to have its roots in the older, Babylonian version.

> In the beginning God created the heaven and the earth. And the earth was without form, and void; and darkness was upon the face of the deep. And the spirit of God moved upon the face of the waters. And God said, Let there be light: and there was light. And God saw the light, that it was good: and God divided the light from the darkness.[15]

Chaos and Consciousness

When I first began reading these origin stories, I thought of Chaos as a real geological time. The stories seemed to describe the beginnings of the earth and its features, of the sun, moon, and the galaxies, in short, those bodies of energy and mass that at some point in geological time did not exist. However, it began to dawn on me (there's the metaphor) that the idea of Chaos is also a description of human, or more accurately, prehuman, consciousness.

At one time, our ancestral apes could not see the landscape of the earth, could not recognize the sun and moon, had no name for water. The ancient stories recall a time when our prehuman ancestors could not perceive shape, color, light, depth, distance, as we do, and had no names for them and no fixed sense of their qualities. This state of being, which we call "nature," rules from inside the animal body; emotions, physiological states, estrus, and mating simply happen, they are not up for question, examination, or rearrangement. Seasons change and fur turns white or brown; the animal is moved from within to interaction with life around it, without externalizing much imagery beyond what (considerable amount) the body conveys through gesture, smell, or sound. Although the inner animal life has its own order, its own integration with the whole, its own rationalism, we rely so much on our culture that the preconscious state before our ancestors learned to think outside themselves was a state we now call Chaos, and greatly fear.

When we fall out of external mind as adults, mental and emotional confusion catch us in a whirlpool of broken boundaries and inexpressable emotion, chiefly terror. Autistic children, who fail to hook onto human culture, live in a frightening place before naming. Children never taught to speak may growl, grunt, and scream, but they say no words. Language must be taught; differentiation—of shape, of color, of day from night, sun from moon, land from water, up from down—must be taught.

The process of learning is a process of separation, and most of the major creation stories describe a change of consciousness through separation. The god, or originating principle, is not heaven, earth, or light itself. The originating principle "creates" heaven, earth, light, and dark by separating them, or as some

10

myths describe, the first beings "emerge" from darkness or from a lower world. The act of separating is the act of creation, and also of consciousness, of understanding the imagery, of mental connection.

But how were those connections first made? While myths capture verbally principles of human existence, human actions are the source of those principles, human actions that lead to human comprehension. A myth merely holds the information in a verbal memory; tens of thousands of years of repeated actions may go into the making of a single line of its story. Fortunately human actions from times prior to ours have been recorded in ethnography, especially in those accounts gathered before Christianization and other religious and moral views (including feminism) required and enabled an end to some of the more dramatic ritual practices of humankind. Disciplined separation is clearly a major factor of human culture, and the most complex and fundamental separation practice is that of first menstruation, or as it is more formally termed, menarche.

Separating Dark from Light

Menstrual seclusion rites as recorded over the last few centuries typically include three basic taboos: the menstruating woman must not see light, she must not touch water, and she must not touch the earth. Since these same elements are differentiated in Genesis and other creation stories, I began to see how menstrual rites might have "created the world" for ancient peoples, and to wonder whether the sleepers who awoke and saw landscape, who named the elements, who separated the above from the below, and darkness from light, were informed by rites of seclusion that specified these very elements, singled them out for attention through *tapua,* sacred law of "the woman's friend."

Human perception began, many creation stories say, when we could distinguish between light and dark. That distant ancestral eyes didn't have the perception of this distinction is easier to com-

11

prehend (how could they not see light?) if we remember that until very recently a person could walk for weeks in dense forest without seeing the sky as more than fragments of glitter through a maze of moving leaves. Not only the equatorial girdle, but much of the Northern Hemisphere was covered with dense forest in the age immediately preceding our own; even the stark sand of the Sahara is believed to have once been forested.

In many parts of a dense forest, light never reaches the ground; it "lives" scattered in the trees, and in constant motion. A band of primates, held to a small forested area by predators and the need for leafy food, lived in a small world, one that didn't need to know the original sources of water or light, merely the keen inner senses to locate water and see with light. For it isn't that the remote ancestors didn't see light, but they saw *with* light, as naturally as breathing. They did not see light as outside of themselves, as having a distinct source, a single place from whence it emanated. They had no origin story of light. Once externalized light was recognized by someone, was perceived as a separate entity, how could she retain and remember it, given that prehumans by definition had no language, no marking system, nothing that we call physical culture. How could they establish noninstinctual knowledge outside of their own bodies? How did we acquire orderly minds of external measurement?

Anthropologists currently believe that the oldest continuous religion on earth is among Australian aborigines, who have a deity named Rainbow Snake. According to legend, two sisters, the Wawilak Sisters, were the first to be swallowed by the Snake. This happened on the occasion when the older sister was giving birth; the younger sister began to dance while they waited for the afterbirth, and suddenly she began her first blood flow. At this instant, the Snake came out of the waterhole, and wrapped itself around both of them and their newborn child. Chris Knight has hypothesized that the Rainbow Snake, coming from the womb of the waterhole, and said to "swallow" a woman when she menstruates, is based in menstrual synchrony, evidently so central to these people that "menstrual blood of three women" is a topic of women's cats-cradle games, and most rituals include "menstrual" flows.[16]

Acquiring an externally based mind required early humans to connect to something outside of themselves as a frame of reference, to connect physically; and this was accomplished when the females evolved a menstrual cycle capable of synchronous rhythm, or *entrainment*. Entrainment is the quality of two similarly timed beats to link up and become synchronized in each other's presence. Non-digital clocks behave this way, and so do drums.[17] This quality of interactive rhythm, being not mechanical, applies as well to the periodicity of menstruation. As has been demonstrated by women volunteers and observers, menstrual periods are highly affected by the environment. Periods are easily disrupted by changes of light, travel through time zones, and severe exercise or dietary deprivation. Menstruation is a malleable cycle, but menstrual periodicity is also able to entrain; women living together and in similar circumstances will often spontaneously synchronize their periods with each other and evidently with any light source that imitates the moon's dark and light cycles. Menstruation has been disrupted by the urban environment, with its irregular lighting.[18] The flexibility of menstrual cycles, their ability to entrain to another regular rhythm, gave ancestral females the inner tool to entrain with other females enough to notice the commonality of blood flow, and to entrain with the moon closely enough to notice it as a source of light and to differentiate its effect from darkness.

This unique cycle in correspondence with the cycles of an outside body, the waxing and waning of the moon far beyond the surface of the earth, taught humans to see from outside of their animal bodies, and to display that knowledge externally, in physical culture. The menstrual mind, became externalized because females were forced to teach its perspective to members of the family who did not menstruate. Males, in learning the pattern, greatly extended it, rearranged it, demonstrated their comprehension one

13

further step, and mirrored back to the females: an ongoing dance of mind between the genders. The consequences of the menstrual/lunar correspondence is what has divided us, for good and ill, from the other animals. Unlike our simian relatives, unlike any other creature, humans use external measurement, the gift of menstruation. We have a lunar/menstrual lever that enables us to move our senses back and forth between the subjective and the objective, and to embody our ideas in external form.

When during the hundreds of thousands of times the ancestral prehumans secluded themselves during what was at least some of the time a collective menstruation at the dark of the moon, they noticed that the light was also hiding. They may also have come to notice that the light at times (dawn) was the same color as their blood. While they were menstruating, they noticed darkness was different from light. Darkness thus had a source: menstruation. At the end of each menstruation, they "created" light when they emerged from darkness, from hiding. And to continue its remembrance and to reinforce the principle, they began emerging from seclusion exactly at dawn, emerging "into the light." They synchronized with darkness and light. And because of the back-and-forth road that is cause and effect, since menstruation "created" light as it "created" dark, so it could also destroy them. The menstruant, especially at menarche, was not allowed to look at light—lest in her condition she destroy it, allowing her society to fall back into Chaos. Menstrual separation was the first step to differentiating light from darkness, and of displaying and remembering the knowledge.

Perhaps this is part of the memory kept alive by seclusion rites recorded in the nineteenth century, which almost universally included a prohibition against seeing light:

> Among the Indians of California a girl at her first menstruation was thought to be possessed of a particular degree of supernatural power, and this was not always regarded as entirely defiling or malevolent. Often, however, there was a strong feeling of the power of evil inherent in her condition. Not only was she secluded from her family and

the community, but an attempt was made to seclude the world from her. One of the injunctions most strongly laid upon her was not to look about her. She kept her head bowed and was forbidden to see the world and the sun. Some tribes covered her with a blanket.[19]

Among many tribes, the menstruant could not see the moon or the sun and had to be covered even when she left the hut at night. In particular, her head and eyes had to be shielded from the great lights in the sky.

How terrifying the first ventures into separation must have been, for at the very beginning of the changes from primate to human, archaeologically dated at around four and a half million years ago, there were *no words* to describe the vision. Wordlessly, a more conscious female pulled her sisters into seclusion with her. Wordlessly, they pushed their daughters into seclusion at the first sign of their blood. Wordlessly, they sat in the moonless night and "saw" darkness as a different state than light. They named it with the act of separation. They "saw" that when anyone menstruating was absent from the group, so was the night light. In this seeing, they perceived light and dark as different states. They saw that light, like the menstruant, separates, and then emerges.

With the act of sitting together in the dark, the early women entered a new world of consciousness. Their minds became "human" through an externalized vision that had as yet and perhaps for millennia to come no other expression than menstrual separation, the creation of consciousness by distinguishing menstruation from other activities. This separation endowed both menstruation and light with power, the power of memory and first cause, the power of rite to create human mind and culture.

The fundamental connection between separation and creation comes through in languages that developed much later, in the word "sacred," which means "set apart" (it also means "curse"), and in the word "sabbath," or *sabbat,* which can be translated as "the divider." The ancient European religion of the goddess Diana celebrated four separations, or Sabbats, as divisions of the year. "Wherever the ancient cult of Diana was extant, its votaries met four times a year to celebrate the mysteries of their faith, and these gatherings, which were known as Sabbats or Sabbaths, were the very heart of their existence as a corporate society."[20]

The original meaning of the Sabbath can be understood as "menstrual separation," particularly as related to the new moon. As the seventh day, it is also "the day of rest" of the Genesis creation story, which took place in seven days—so each week is a re-creation of the Beginning. The number of days of menstrual seclusion is specified for Hebrew women in Leviticus 15:19, and it is seven. Menstrual seclusion is implied as well in the Babylonian creation myth, the oldest one known, which lists in its sixth line, after descriptions of Tiamat and Apsu, a special kind of sacred reed hut, the *giparu*, which I take to be a menstrual seclusion hut.[21]

When the ancestress of four and a half million years ago separated in the earliest Sabbats, she stepped out of Chaos, and across a terrifying abyss of mind. What makes the Abyss so ominous is that to enter human mind we step out of the security of instinct, the net of animal mind, and enter the frail social construct of a rite, which is only held in place externally and accessed through cultural memory and repetition. The farther we get from inner knowledge, the more dependent on the external mind we become. The Abyss yawned before those who did not keep the separation, for in their newfound understanding they established a principle correspondence: without menstrual separation, there *was* no light. Menstrual seclusion rites continually created light and separated it from dark. Without menstrual separation and the emphasis taboo placed on the seeing of light, the idea of light having a source would have flickered and gone out. And probably, many times, it did.

By using *tapua*, women were able to hold the thought still, to capture the perception of the source of light, emphasize its importance, and teach it. Every time a girl began her period for the first time, she separated and was not allowed to see light. Then at the end of her bleeding, she emerged into the light. "After a girl emerges from seclusion, the . . . women take her around and show her the earth, bodies of water, flowers, trees—as though she is see-

16

ing them for the first time."[22] In this way, seclusion reenacts the original awakening of human consciousness.

In a typical seclusion, on the occasion of her first menstruation, which is called "entrance into the shade," or *Chol Mlop,* a Khmer girl in Cambodia was secluded in a darkened, curtained-off section of the house; she was forbidden to look upon men and allowed to go outdoors only in the dark night. The "shade" lasted several months, sometimes as long as a year, and during this time she learned skills of weaving and basketmaking. The end of her cloistering, called "coming out of the shade," featured a feast with relatives and friends, who made offerings to ancestors and spirits, as well as a number of rites similar to those for weddings.[23]

Separate huts were often built so that the initiates could not see light: "Among the Yaracares, an Indian tribe of Bolivia, at the eastern foot of the Andes, when a girl perceives the signs of puberty, her father constructs a little hut of palm leaves near the house."[24] "When a Hindu maiden reaches maturity she is kept in a dark room for four days, and is forbidden to see the sun. . . . Similarly among the Parivarams of Madura, when a girl attains to puberty she is kept for sixteen days in a hut, which is guarded at night by her relations."[25]

Menstrual seclusion rites reenacted their own discoveries, returning women back along a path of unraveling time, to the chaotic mind before light was seen. Menstrual seclusion accomplished this by a simple taboo: the menstruant was not allowed to see light. On the North American continent, she had to cover her head with a deerskin before going outdoors and was shut away in a dark place for days, even weeks, at a time; in Southeast Asia, she might have been wrapped in a hammock or shut up in a little hut or a square of mats, or she had to lie down in the dark part of a house for days and nights on end. Silence often accompanied the cloistering; she could not speak, or she could not speak above a whisper, or her name could not be spoken during the sacred time—as though she was returning deliberately to a preconscious state.

The reasons given for this and the other menstrual taboos were

17

that harm would come to the menstruant; she would sicken or die, her bones would break, she would become infertile. But some peoples held taboos in which the menstruant's destructive power affected all life and even the features of the landscape. If a woman broke taboo, not only would she herself be harmed, but harm would come to others, to her family, her village. Her eyes had special power; she could not look at others or they would sicken. She could not drop blood on the path, for someone might step on it and later die or be infertile. She had to avoid talking to her husband or touching his weapons lest harm befall him in the hunt; she was forbidden to cross the path of a hunting party. She was sexually dangerous, harm would come to any partner's genitals, and person, so she could not have sex. If she failed to keep her taboos, her community would no longer thrive. Thus, she could not look at the sky or the planets. Nor could she gaze at bodies of water, for fear of causing a flood; if she were to look at trees and plants, they would wither. She had to protect the sources of water, so she could not look at the pond, or it would dry up. Her glance would cause the village cows to sicken and die, or their milk to dry up; it caused crops to wither in the fields. She had, in her blood rites taken as a whole, complete power over all that humans depend on for their lives, all we had deciphered about the universe—for, as I have argued, it was menstrual consciousness that first created all these elements. And so many of the rites involved silence, as though they were laid down during the long eras before speech, when action alone did the creating.

Hers was the power of raveling and of unraveling, since what consciousness (spirit, mystery, and mind) gives us, it can also take back. And the power of creation and destruction, as at one time evidently all humanity believed, was in the woman's blood.

Metaphor and Metaform

As a poet, I work with the power of metaphor and with its mechanics, and I have long been aware that metaphor isn't just a method of description. Some metaphors are so powerful they become translated into physical form. If a poem emphatically states (with believable graphic details) that a woman is a rattlesnake, some of the power of the "snake" to strike in its own behalf is transferred to the cultural idea "woman." A metaphor is a figure of speech using measurement, comparison, for the purpose of transferring power; in this example the power of a real rattlesnake may be assumed by a real woman. If repeated use of this snake poem leads a woman to take a self-defense class, for example, she then converts the poetic metaphor into a *form*. In the class she may even learn to strike two fingers in her attacker's eyes "like a snake's fangs." In a different context, a chanted poem using the metaphor of a woman as a snake might accompany a dance in which a young woman learns to twine her arms, legs, and trunk in sinewy "snake" movements; perhaps she also wears the tail of a rattler as a bracelet that makes a rhythmic sound as she dances. In both cases, the women are altering their own bodies in ways that originate with real beings, rattlesnakes.

Historically human culture, as we shall see, has used such creatures for all kinds of purposes. In examining the power of verbal metaphor, I began to see that we surround ourselves with living, interacting, physically *embodied* metaphors. And in tracing the use of such physical forms as comparisons, as measurement, I found that remarkable numbers of everyday objects, artifacts, creatures, and human cultural habits can be traced back, through mythology and anthropology, to a single element of measurement: menstruation. My search for women's contribution to science and culture has thus intersected with my poetic explorations of how metaphor translates into genuine cultural power.

Our menstrual-minded ancestress stepped out of her excellent net of animal intelligence into the potentially chaotic external mind, the mind unique to human beings. The human mind uses metaphoric imagery, what I call "external measurement." Our originators could not have stepped across the Abyss without simultaneously finding a way to hold the first few ideas in place, since they disappear in the absence of culture. Neither instinct nor the central nervous system store such imagery. It has to be externalized, and it is fragile. It has to be taught; and to be taught, it has to be remembered. This required techniques resembling metaphor but much more extreme; the metaphor somehow had to be actualized, acted out in the physical.

Our ancestresses taught via menstrual instruction, through rituals that embodied ideas based on menstrual information. I call this *metaform*, specifically, *an act or form of instruction that makes a connection between menstruation and a mental principle.* At first I thought to call the forms that menstruation creates *menstruaforms,* but that seemed too narrow a word for what I mean. I chose metaform instead, meaning a physical embodiment of metaphor in which menstruation is one part of the equation. *Meta* means among, with, after, and also change, and I like its implication of transformative measurement: measured form, metaform. I also like the sense of a super- or panvision, as in *meta*physics, though I don't mean "beyond the physical." A metaform is an idea that translates into physical form, and conversely, it is also the physical form that embodies or "holds" an idea, with menstruation as its source. My broadest (and ultimately unprovable) premise is that all metaphor, all measurement, and all cultural forms, could they be traced back far enough, would lead us to menstruation and menstrual rite.

If—as we are told in a multitude of creation stories—the act that enabled the human mind to emerge from Chaos was an act of separation, then menstrual seclusion rites are repeated separations consisting of metaforms that contain creation stories.

Chaos is forgetting learned metaphoric patterns, forgetting metaformic instruction. And since our original millions-of-years-ago ancestress presumably was completely of the animal world, she could take only one step out of that fully developed order, only one step at a time away from the network of animal interactions that maintained the pattern of her life, and of her family's life. She had as yet no language, no poetry, no drawing, no masks or music with

20

which to convey her first external insight. She had only the intelligence of her own body and its actions; she had only her blood, and its peculiar entrainment with the moon. And when she secluded herself in imitation of the moon, she externalized the metaphoric connection.

We now think in metaphors, and we think *with* metaphors, as molds into which we pour the stuff of everyday experience. But we get these metaphoric molds, these meta*forms,* not from blind imagination, but from our very specific and historic interactions with the external and internal physical world, remembered through rites and ceremonies handed down to us—by now, through dozens of channels. The original metaforms were set in place millions of years before humans had speech, and they were based in the synchrony inherent in the menstrual cycle, as well as in the ability of the primate mind to think in terms of mimicry and metaphor.

Metaphor itself is a form of synchronicity, measuring the inner with the outer. Metaphor says that one thing is another; it says they are entrained through repetition of pattern. Metaphor measures through comparison. The recognition of similarity and dissimilarity of category between elements is how we think, and the external expression of this recognition is what makes us human. The transformation of such an idea into a metaform, an external expression of the synchronization of two patterns, is what enables human communication. Metaform transforms one thing into another, endowing two unlike things with equality of power, in our minds.

As biological science tells us, though the animals continue to evolve, the interactions, skills, and intelligence of nonhuman beings appears to have achieved ecological balance—a sustainable economy. Their nonhuman minds appear to be perfect for what they set out to do. What disrupts this ecological balance are the extreme actions of humankind; consequently, we appear in our ways of being to be unfinished—still struggling mightily, especially with ourselves. We differ from the animal mind, from what Western biology calls "instinct," in that animal minds are almost en-

21

tirely inner. Though we still have instincts, cultural teachings and misteachings can completely disrupt them. We have become dependent on our external minds.

We have constructed our minds externally, not abstractly, but through using physical metaphors—metaforms—that embody a comparison to a menstrually based idea. Two good examples of metaforms are the chair and the hut. These forms are so culturally ingrained that virtually any adult stranded at length in the wilderness could construct, from memory, a rude hut and some version of a chair. As we shall see, both "chair" and "hut" are rooted in menstrual rite.

Metaforms are physical, mental, and also spiritual. By spirit I mean that metaforms at times "speak" to us in some fashion, and people understand this communication as a dialogue with a non-human intelligent spirit, or deity, as messages from the mind of the cosmos. Nonmaterialist peoples have had terms that combine all three spheres, for example the Maori word *aria,* meaning a spirit that enters—say, a snake—and conveys a message to humans.[26] The Bible and other mythology refer to speaking huts, walls, and thrones; rocks, plants, and animals speak to tribal and psychic folk; and psychiatrists work with the divinatory nature of dreams, whose images speak to us of our deepest comprehensions of life. My contention is that the central unit of measurement, the ultimate metaphor, to which all metaforms refer, is blood.

To help sort through the varieties of metaform, I have divided them into four categories, corresponding to the ways human society has remembered, taught, and acted out menstrual principles. Logically, the first of these seems to have been *wilderness* metaform: the use of creatures, formations, and elements of nature to describe menstrual ideas. The second is *cosmetic* metaform, for which the Greek word *cosmetikos* seems appropriate, with its dual meanings of "a sense of harmony and order" and "one skilled in adorning," from *cosmos,* meaning both "ornament" and "the universe as a well-ordered whole." Expanding on this, I use *cosmetic* metaform to mean the ordering of the world through descriptive use of human body action, artful movement, shape, ornament and decoration, and even ingestion of meaningful foods. Third is *narrative* metaform, based in language, sound, number, and story, which came about as people imagined themselves and their originators to be characters in a life cycle. Fourth is *material* metaform, characteristic of our current civilization: the separation of spirit from matter, and the use of earth's being to craft products into forms expressive of current external ideas.

Chapter 2

Light Moved on the Water

T H E ancestral menstruant who crouched in a tree or on the ground in a bower of boughs, hiding from predatory teeth, was connected to darkness because her period was so often entrained with the dark of the moon. Darkness, death, fear, silence—all remain connected in many cultures. The menstruant's many taboos not to see light also connected her to light, into which she emerged in triumph at the end of her period. Her blood was analogous as well to water, so that all water was comprehended in terms of menstrual flow, as we know from the myth of Rainbow Snake, which equates the collective sisterly vaginal snake to various waters in the sky and on the ground. The menstruant's blood flow must not mingle with the earth's "blood" flow lest Chaos, loss of consciousness in the form of a flood, annihilate human life. Her world-forming "waters" had to be separated from nature's "waters."

This separation of various liquids created them as distinct natural forms with the characteristics of the body—bodies of water. Streams were understood as having a single source, like menstrual blood flowing from the vulva spring. Springs, pools, and mountain lakes were endowed with sacred character, dread, and taboo. To tribal people in what is now Oregon, Crater Lake was considered the most sacred spot, the center of the earth, and none but a select few were ever allowed to look upon it. (Even in modern times, Crater Lake retains a treacherous reputation.) In England, wells and springs still bear pagan female names such as "Maiden's Well" or "Bride's Spring."

Menstrual seclusion rite enacted the creation of the world and its elements, forming them as conscious ideas before there was language or sense of narrative enough to make them into a story; the rites themselves constituted the creation story. The menstruant was tabooed from seeing light, and then her emergence from dark seclusion was directly *into* the light, at dawn, thus bringing light into focus. She was separated from water, and her blood flow was believed to influence the flow of bodies of water. Her blood flow was the original comprehension of water, of water as a substance, of water as a moving force capable of causing chaos or death. Our simian ancestress began to perceive water as a mental, rather than an instinctual or strictly physical, reference. The animal perceives water primarily by smell, and though smell remained a part of the mythology of menstruation and water—in the Australian myth, the Rainbow Snake smells blood and causes a flood—gradually the sense of smell as a means of identification of water was replaced with sight, the visual perception of different kinds of water, and of bodies of water as entities, related to other kinds of water, yet distinctly themselves. These distinctions were enacted repeatedly through menstrual rite and the tabooed approaches of the menstruant toward forms of water.

The Proto- or All-Moon and the Separation of Waters

The apparently simple act of separating the movement of the moon in the sky from the movement of the reflection of the moon on bodies of water must have taken millennia, perhaps hundreds of thousands or millions of years. Many myths mention light moving on the water or the separating of the waters. I once tracked the reflection of the moon across tidal inland waters far below my seat in an airplane on the coast of the eastern United States. For about ten minutes, the moon was clearly and intermittently reflected, twenty or thirty thousand feet below me. The effect was startling

25

and eerie, even frightening, because I did not recognize it as the moon. I saw the light, large, sprawling, and beautiful, and kept trying to identify it as a beam from the plane or some other industrial source. "What *is* that light," I said to myself, finally looking up and noticing the moon in the sky. In the absence of being told by my culture that the larger, rippling light below was a reflection of the smaller more contained light above, I would never have guessed the improbable, that the smaller, stiller light was causing the larger, more fluid one—let alone could I possibly have guessed that both are reflections of the sun.

According to many origin stories, people could not distinguish between the moon and the sun for a very long time after separating light from dark. According to the OED, the roots of the word "light" lead back to the moon, not to the sun: from the root Aryan *leuk,* meaning both "white" and "to shine"; also *loukua,* "moon"; Latin *lucere,* "to shine," and *luna,* "moon"; Old Irish *luan,* "moon"; Welsh *llug,* "light"; and Old slavic, *luca,* "beam of light." Both Lugh and Lucifer were old names for the god of light as connected to the moon.[1] In the beginning, people thought all light had the same source, they saw moon and sun as the same body, an all-moon, or protomoon. They did not separate the sun into its own source with its own cycle until relatively recently—perhaps less than ten thousand years ago.

The people of Ntomba in Zaïre say that before the hero Mokele went upstream by boat and found the sun hidden in a cave, "there was no sunshine yet, there was only moonshine, and the people of Ntomba called the moon the sun!"[2] In much of Africa, moon worship prevailed until recent centuries. People in Uganda have a myth explaining why the moon is ruler: because the moon "arrived first" before the sun did.[3] In Genesis, light and dark were distinguished before the moon and sun were. In many myths, the moon is created long before the sun, sometimes a generation or two before. The Sumerian genealogy of creation gods lists Mammu ("great waters") and An/Ki, (sky/earth), as the first generation, followed by deities of air and reeds in the marsh. The third generation of gods includes the moon as a male and female pair, Nanna and Ningal; and not until the fourth generation, is the sun, Umash, named as son of the moon couple. The moon, in this myth, gave birth to the sun.[4] In Greek myth, too, Apollo the sun is child of Leto, the moon.

According to many creation stories, after light and dark were differentiated, the next act of perception was the separation of the waters from each other, the distinguishing of the different kinds of water, and the naming of water as an element necessary for life. Differentiation of the different kinds of water as variations of the same substance was an enormous task, but according to Genesis it had to be (was) accomplished before dry earth was established. For many, many peoples, including those of Mesopotamia who first formed biblical mythology, the sky was made of water, or was a firmament—a bank—that held back the water, keeping the stuff from falling all at one time. From a menstrual point of view, the "spirit of God" that moved on the waters in the Genesis myth was the all-moon, reflected in the waters on the earth and moving across the waters of the sky as a single entity, the same being making the journey over and over.

It was the menstruant who had the power to cause and, through regulating her behavior, prevent flooding:

> Once upon a time [as the Toba tell]; a woman was menstruating. Her mother and sister forgot to leave drinking water for her. So she went down to the lagoon to drink. It rained until all the people were drowned. All the corpses turned into birds and flew up. . . . This is because Rainbow is angry when a menstruating woman goes near a lagoon.[5]

How the woman's power was woven into ideas of spirits of water is evident in the following example from the Tiwi people of Melville Island, from information gathered by Jane C. Goodale, of rites occurring around 1950. With a girl's first blood, she achieved a special status, called *murinaleta*, that lasted four menstrual periods.

> During her first menstrual period the *murinaleta* is removed from the general camp and makes a new camp in the bush with a number of other women. Her companions usually include her mother, her

co-wives, and any other senior women in her residential group. No
men are allowed in this camp. . . . She cannot touch any water, even
in a container, but must wait for someone to lift the container to her
lips, for otherwise she would fall ill. . . . She cannot look at bodies
of salt or fresh water, for the *maritji* might be angered and come and
kill her. The *maritji* are spirit beings who have a body like a goanna
or "quiet" crocodile. There are many of these spirits, men, women,
and children, and they come in many colors. Their *imunka* (souls)
are like rainbows. A big rainbow is likely to be the *imunka* of a
woman and child *maritji*. The *maritji* are to be treated carefully, for
they can kill a person or they can cause a great "sea" to rise up and
destroy the land. They live in swamps at various localities throughout the two islands, and generally, if treated with respect and caution, will not harm the local inhabitants. Menstruating and pregnant
women and new-born infants, however, are considered to be very
vulnerable to the dangers of the *maritji* and, therefore, must take
extra precautions and completely avoid the homes of the *maritji*.

 These taboos and several others such as keeping silent, not being
seen by her husband, not scratching her skin apply only to the first
period of menses, but . . . "a woman must observe several lesser
precautions during her monthly periods." These include not going
near small bodies of water, lest they dry up. She must not take long
trips over salt water or the *maritji* will blow up a storm.[6]

The separation of the menstruant from water while in her hut or
other seclusion area was carried to meticulous extreme. In all her
menstrual rites, she was not permitted to leave seclusion and go to
water but drank from a special container, brought to her in her
"shade" by female attendants. Some families kept menstrual drinking cups that passed from generation to generation, never used for
any other purpose; others destroyed the container after each separation.[7] In more than one tribe, the menstruant could only drink
through a straw made of the wing bone of a swan. In an Eskimo
tradition, the bone was that of a white-headed eagle. For other
peoples, the menstruant's drinking straw had to be made from the
leg bone of a crane, goose, or swan. If we think of the woman's
flesh as a metaphor for earth, and the white bird as a metaphor for
moon or clouds, and the water for sky, then in the very act of her

drinking, the straw leg bone by its own origins served to separate the two elements.

For the most part, the menstruant could not wash during seclusion, even if her rites lasted weeks, but upon her emergence she was required to wash. In some rites, her mother or other attendants came to wash her. Although I have been told there is no prohibition against swimming during menstruation, Jewish tradition retains the sense of separation between ritually clean and unclean: "Among the Jews, the medium of purification was known as 'the water of separation,' the latter term being that used in reference to the menstrual seclusion of women."[8] Orthodox Jewish women still take the ritual end-of-menstruation bath, the *mikveh*.

After fire and steam were added to rites, the menstruant often could not drink cold water, it had to be warm. There are many examples of the necessity to drink only warm water in seclusions among California Indian tribes of the nineteenth century, and remnants of the older extremes remain in practice even where the seclusion rites have died out. In villages in Portugal today, menstruating women avoid cold beverages.[9] And my own women friends have always advised me to drink warm tea during my period as a cure for cramping, and so of course I advise it also: Stay in bed, drink warm soothing tea, let your mind drift where it will. The waters, in menstrual seclusion, are effectively separated.

"Don't go swimming or get wet when you have your period," girls in my junior high in 1953 warned each other. Meanwhile, in health and hygiene classes, the instructors read pamphlets and showed films stressing the modern idea of menstruation, describing it repeatedly as "normal," and giving advice meant to undo older prohibitions held in the folk culture without directly acknowledging that they existed: "You will not be harmed by swimming during your period." The films and pamphlets showed girls swimming, playing sports, smiling, having a wonderful time, as though menstruation equaled summer vacation. Menstruation was, according to the hygiene class, a minor inconvenience easily solved with napkins. Later, tampons would compete as the product of choice for the modern woman, though when they first appeared, the girls I knew all believed they weren't for virgins. They would harm us, we thought. The nature of the harm was vague; we did not know the word hymen.

My first lover, Yvonne, was three years into college and still telling me wide-eyed that a friend had died of a wasting disease years after breaking the menstrual taboo restricting activity. "She used to go swimming and even horseback riding during her period, and everyone said she would die if she kept it up, and then she did! She died because she didn't listen to the older women!" No quoting from hygiene handbooks persuaded her that the truism she had heard as a girl in the back country of New Mexico was anything but accurate advice. I don't know if the source of this taboo belief was the Spanish tradition brought to the region in the sixteenth century, local Indian belief, or a teaching of Yvonne's Polish-born mother. It could have been from any of them, given that Yvonne was repeating one of the oldest and most widely held seclusion beliefs.

As we saw from the Tiwi example, the prohibition against touching water was for the protection of the people as a whole. It marked the ability of human minds to remember, predict, and fear storms, floods, the destructive force of water, as well as its life-giving properties, which must—by human endeavor—be protected. It was also a reminder that rain washes out trails—how, if instinct and smell failed, could the earliest humans find each other again, find home base, if water wiped out the trail? The terrors of flood have always been associated with Chaos.

World Formation Story: The Great Flood

For some peoples, the formation of earth as a solid place was the result of an ancestral "fall" from above: In the beginning there was only the spirit world. Women lived in the watery sky, and the earth did not exist. In some accounts, all the people lived in the sky and then fell to earth. In others, the women threw a loop around the moon to climb on, and one who was heavily pregnant fell down to earth, and so we all must now live on earth. The world was all of a piece with few boundaries. Then the ancestress fell out of the watery sky, and her landing created solid earth and greater differentiation of the world's dimensions.

In the Iroquois version of earth creation, Falling Woman falls or is pushed through a hole in the Sky World; below her stretches an endless sea. Water birds rise to break her fall. They help her onto Turtle's back. Diving for mud, the birds heap it onto Turtle's back, and the earth is thus formed. Turtle, with its square shell and four table legs, is a metaform for earth, floating in water as does the earth in old cosmogonies.

Most peoples of the ancient world imagined earth as an island or strip of solid ground floating on the sea. Given that water and the sky are the same color, that the sky, mountains, and the moon are reflected in lakes, that waterdrops on leaves reflect and resemble the light in the sky, how *did* humans acquire a definition of solid earth? How, in the absence of instinct about direction, did they acquire the orientation that directed summer and winter migrations, that allowed gathering and hunting troops to find their way back to "home camp," that enabled people living near rivers that yearly overflow to seek higher ground before disaster drowned every single one? How did they express that orientation externally, so it could be remembered and passed along the generations? The Flood can be described as loss of consciousness, overwhelming mental as well as physical chaos, the quality of being "lost." The Flood myth, in all its permutations, is surely the most universal of the ancient stories.

As recently as the mid 1900s, storytellers in the Scottish Highlands had witches raising storms by means of thread and water bowls. One method of capsizing a particular ship was to put a small vessel to float in a bowl of milk or water. Through incantations, the liquid was caused to whirl in a lunar direction until the little vessel capsized, and simultaneously, the big ship on the real sea would be capsized in a sudden storm. This alleged power of the

31

sorceror woman is of course straight out of the menstrual hut with its containment of her flood capacity by separation of her person from water through use of special bowls and straws. According to Frazer, menstruating women were not allowed to travel in boats lest they inadvertently cause a storm.[10] The stormy power of the individual witch, shaman, or sorceror transferred to the collective creator/destroyer goddess in narratives.

A few myths make an explicit connection between the Flood and menstruation: The Wemale people tell of the sun god Tuwale causing a great flood. His daughter Bouwa stops it by covering her vulva with a silver girdle for three days. This act (of *cosmetikos*) stops the flood, and since then women menstruate for three days.[11]

Some Flood myths use the metaform of the Snake, the great external vagina who swallows bleeding women: The Wawilak Sisters of Arnhem Land, the elder one bleeding from the afterbirth and the younger one menstruating for the first time, approach a water hole owned by the female rock python, Julunggul. She smells blood and makes lightning and rain, washing some afterbirth blood into the pool. The aroused python follows the sisters to their "shade," pushes the door open, and swallows them. When she returns to her pool, she talks to the other pythons, and then the whole countryside is flooded. In another version, of the Murngin, the python Yurlunggur is male, his title being "Big Father." He smells the blood when it trickles into his pool, and as he advances toward the sisters, who sing to keep him back, a flood precedes him.[12]

The drama of keeping humanity safe, conscious, and in some measure of control over the elemental forces around them is made very clear in the male role of Medatia, in a myth told among tribal people in the south of Venezuela. The shaman Medatia works to restore his people's memories. The men have been killed, and the women have been stolen by the *mawadi,* who live in the river, taking the form of anacondas.

> Then Medatia went into the waters and rapids and came to Huiio, the great snake's house where she lives with her *mawadi* people. We see Huiio and the *mawadi* as anaconda. Sometimes we see Huiio as the rainbow. She brings us rain and harvests. She also brings our

children sickness. Medatia found many women there and because he had *wiriki,* little crystals that let him "see inside," he prompted them to remember who they really were and that they did not belong to the *mawadi.* The women listened, fell asleep and dreamed, and returned to their own houses on Earth. "We remember it all now," they said, "We woke up." They remembered how the *mawadi* came out of the rapids, made them pregnant, killed the men, and brought hurricanes destroying everything. Then another woman said, "We were gathering water in gourds by the edge of the river. I was very young. Suddenly blood started coming out. It was my first blood. The *mawadi* smelled it down there in their house in the water. When the blood fell in the river, they were crazy with desire. They came up from below in droves. They flooded the banks and our house. They took us down in the water."

That's why now, the men shut their women up away from the rivers and the houses when they menstruate. That's so the *mawadi* don't find them; so they don't take them away or flood the houses.[13]

Rainbow Snake is aroused when menstrual water gets into lagoon water. This mixing of vital waters makes the god(dess) of synchronous consciousness, Rainbow Snake, angry. Chaos, the complete destruction of landscape and all humanity, is the result. People cannot remember where they live. Separation of the waters is essential to maintain the orientation of people to location, to dry land. Conscious memory is maintained through the separation of menstrual blood, the fundamental life water. The institution of menstrual seclusion and menstrual consciousness enabled people to recognize the distinct nature of water in its various forms, as something "other" than the element "earth."

The original covenant the people make with Snake is that menstrual blood will not get into the water; the menstruant will seclude herself and will be extremely careful about separating her body fluids, not only her blood but even the spit of her mouth, from touching water. The men, through the crossover office of shamanism, will understand the necessity for the seclusion rites by assisting in maintaining them. The Snake keeps its side of the covenant by staying in the sky clearly and safely visible as the rainbow marking the end of a storm. "You see me," Snake says by this display, "so

33

you know I am not chasing you, and you know there is no threat of flood." Human mind, with its memory, orientation, and orderly recognition of the elements, is thus held in place by proper menstrual rite, and the chaos of Flood is held at bay.

Of the great variation of flood myths from around the world, most have no direct reference to menstruation. But many include snakes and blood; many others have as main characters wilderness metaforms, such as birds, dogs, or coyotes, that are connected to menstruation in other myths. For example, in Navajo and other Native American stories, Coyote—the originator of menstruation—causes a flood. In South America, a dog, often a black dog, locates dry land after the flood. It comes back muddy, so the people know land is appearing again. A number of flood stories use body fluids other than blood—urine, tears, or spit—in a continual fine-splitting of our waters. The color red is frequently present. In one South American myth, the flood is the result of mutilating a red parrot.

In many stories, the primary characters climb trees to escape the waters or climb to the tops of mountains. While this must be in part a reference to actual behavior, the persistent myth is clearly not just about the instinct to flee water by dashing to higher ground. If it were, people would simply do the running or climbing, they would not develop rituals and stories about it. The tree stops the mental, culturally chaotic Flood because the light in the sky visible from the top of the tree can be used for orientation; or the tree is the tallest and can itself be used for orientation; or the mountain is the site of lunar or stellar rituals and observations that establish orientation. In one North American tale, a woman causes a flood and is later turned into the moon. In one of the Arnhem Land myths, the humans are rescued by the morning star—a light body used to mark time of the night and time of the year.

World Creation Taboos and Land

According to the creation sequence in Genesis, first light and dark were differentiated and then the various kinds of water were sepa-

34

rated, so that the sky was designated as one source of water, and bodies of water below were designated as another. Thus water was "gathered into one place" and perceived, or named, as a lake, river, or lagoon. Only then did dry land appear and become designated as "earth." As backward as this sequence appears to our logical minds, it is repeated in creation myths from many cultures. Just as "dark" was comprehended first and then, through the menstrual cycle, came recognition of emerging light, "dry," or earth, could only be defined in contrast to "wet." Earth was not "grounded" as a concept until there was consciousness of water as a discrete substance, and it is to this ancient understanding that the Flood myth refers.

Although the menstruant often was placed in a pit in the earth, in other seclusion rites, she was forbidden to touch the earth. In addition to regulations concerning her relationship to light and to water, the menstruant typically had to follow taboos concerning the earth. She could not get her blood on the earth, or touch the earth: "Thus among the Negroes of Loango girls at puberty are confined in separate huts, and they may not touch the ground with any part of their bare body." [14] Sometimes this prohibition was effected by huts or other devices that kept her raised up off the earth: "In New Ireland girls are confined for four or five years in small cages, being kept in the dark and not allowed to set foot on the ground." [15] A hammock slung from a house top or tree was often used in South America: "When symptoms of puberty appeared on a girl for the first time, the Guaranis of Southern Brazil, on the borders of Paraguay, used to sew her up in her hammock, leaving only a small opening in it to allow her to breathe. In this condition, wrapt up and shrouded like a corpse, she was kept for two or three days or so long as the symptoms lasted, and during this time she had to observe a most rigorous fast." [16]

Sometimes not touching the earth was specified for other parts of menstrual rite besides the period of seclusion. In New Guinea, following a seclusion of five days and two months of various taboos, the emerging menstruant was carried down the household ladder on her grandmother's back. [17] Great attention was paid to

35

keeping the menstruant's body off the earth, even if it required the labor of a number of other women to carry her from place to place on her menstrual route. In James Frazer's account of menstrual rites on the island of Mabuiag, of the Torres Straits, one or two old maternal aunts care for a girl at her menarche: She squats in a heap of bushes up to her head, in a darkened corner of the house, prohibited from seeing the sun; she comes out at night only, she may not handle food and is fed by her attendants. No man may come near her lest his fishing boat later crash. At the end of three months she is "carried down to a freshwater creek by her attendants, hanging on to their shoulders in such a way that her feet do not touch the ground, while the women of the tribe form a ring round her. . . . At the shore, she is stripped of her ornaments, and the bearers stagger with her into the creek, where they immerse her, and all the other women join in splashing water over both the girl and her bearers. When they come out of the water, one of the attendants makes a heap of grass for her charge to squat upon." [18]

In some cultures, the "path" was specified as the area needing protection from the menstruant's dangerous blood. If a girl began to bleed while out in the countryside or village, she had to avoid the path; "Among the Zulus and kindred tribes of South Africa . . . should she be overtaken by the first flow while she is in the fields, she must, after hiding in the bush, scrupulously avoid all pathways in returning home. A reason for this avoidance is assigned by the A-Kamba of British East Africa [Kenya], whose girls under similar circumstances observe the same rule. 'If,' they say, 'a stranger accidently trod on a spot of blood and then cohabited with a member of the opposite sex before the girl was better again, it is believed that she would never bear a child.'" [19] Similar beliefs were reported by many Native Americans, people of the South Pacific, and other places.

In many origin myths, the earth at first was not solid and had no landscape features. Earth when it finally appears after light, dark, and the separated waters, often begins as a bit of mud, as in Iroquois and other Native American stories of earth being piled up, a beakful at a time, by water birds or other creators. Even among people long accustomed to the idea of a large, solid earth, the ground continues to move: anthropologist Marija Gimbutas in a lecture once described people of her native Lithuania believing that rocks move around of their own volition.

We of the materialist world view subscribe to a convention, agreeing to believe that the earth, and matter, are solid. Our physicists tell us otherwise, and so does the cosmology we have inherited from peoples of all regions and ages, for whom place and time are not necessarily fixed. In the absence of clock time, both place and time are relative to interactions with other beings. A mountain seen at a distance at noon when the overhead sun flattens out details seems much farther away than it does at 4 P.M. Even such immediate forms as tree leaves seem much larger when the sun's rays slant. Without fixed ideas about time, mountains "move," trees change shape, the earth "floats." Those of us who have lived around the Pacific region known as the "Rim of Fire" and other earthquake and volcano zones can more easily acknowledge the correctness of the ancestral view: the earth is *not* solid.

When a volcano boils lava and ash, our understanding of the earth as a solid plane melts as the mountain does, or as the giant plates beneath us do when one slides under another. When an earthquake cracks house walls and foundations, splits the earth into deep gullies, and increases the height of nearby mountains by as much as five feet, the idea of a fixed earth is shattered. I once experienced an earthquake outside, and saw the earth of my yard ripple like a horse's back shaking off a fly, so though along with everyone else I speak of "solid ground," I know the expression is an agreed-upon social illusion. From such experiences one can enter the more chaotic minds of our premythic, less materialist ancestors, who lived all their lives without perceiving the earth as solid or as categorically different from water and sky.

Touching Her Body, the Earth

One of the most common regulations in menstrual seclusion rites concerns the menstruant's body. She does not touch others or their property. Often, no one is allowed to touch her; more often still, she is not allowed to touch herself, not allowed to scratch her skin or her head with her fingers.

Menstrual seclusion rites suggest that the method for comprehending and establishing the earth as solid was metaformic, the transfer of understanding the outside of one's own skin as a border to understanding the surface of the earth as skin and therefore border. If the menstruant scratched her skin with her fingers like any other animal, the perception of solidity or surface would disappear. Moreover, she would bleed onto her skin, which would harm it, just as blood touching the earth would harm the earth. In many, many creation myths, the earth is female. The skin of women has long been equated with the surface of the earth, a way of remembering the principle and teaching the metaform.

The ritual perception of solid earth as skin needed a formal practice, one that established distance between finger and skin. The menstruant's nails were, and remain, recognized as instruments capable of drawing blood. In seclusion, she kept her hands away from herself and held them passively. She used a twig to touch herself instead of her finger, and later she carried an elaborately carved special stick, a scratching stick, into her seclusion.

To not touch her own body, to not scratch herself for the duration of menstrual seclusions (which in some tribes and societies could last as long as a month, even years), required great strength of mind, yet this formal practice was rigidly adhered to, and reappears frequently in menstrual rites. The discipline required for this rite alone would create a person in such control of her own body, with such mental concentration, as to give her entirely different capacities than the ape family rootstock, by now far behind her.

Besides not touching, other taboos seem designed to call extreme attention to the surface of the body. In some menarchal rites, the menstruant was lashed with a limb, or flailed with cords "to make her strong" or "to make her fertile." These whippings were not done in anger or as punishment, for otherwise the girl was treated with love and care. The Kitanemuk tribe of the southwestern United States used a particularly painful method:

38

At her first menses a girl was often lashed with nettles by her mother, then washed with hot water containing pounded estafiata (a plant species); she was also given some to drink. . . . Then the girl ran back and forth between two rocks about 150 feet apart, chased by a woman chosen for her industriousness. Next the girl was taken to a small isolated hut constructed by her father. Here she remained for four months with an elderly kinswoman. . . . After the period of confinement the girl was bathed by her mother, and (a number of) restrictions were ended. . . . When her first regular menstruation occurred the girl used a specially constructed scratching stick of wood or abalone shell; she also lay face down on a bed of nettles for three days. At each subsequent menses the girl . . . used the scratching stick for a week. After marriage she used the stick only prior to childbirth.[20]

Being lashed on the outside of her skin with nettles, then lying face down on a bed of them for three days, might have taught distant ancestors of these people, unforgettably, the lesson about surfaces.

A clue about the reasoning behind the taboo against scratching is contained in the following example of a hunter's taboo from the South Seas: "In the island of Nias the hunters sometimes dig pits, cover them over lightly with twigs, grass, and leaves, and then drive game into them. While they are engaged in digging the pits, they have to observe a number of taboos . . . [For example, while they are] *in the pit they may not scratch themselves, for if they did the earth would be loosened and would collapse.*"[21] Having so carefully preserved the earth over who knows how many thousands of generations by keeping the menstruant off the earth, people approached digging with the utmost caution, lest the earth fall apart and the still tender idea of the surface of the earth unravel, merging borders again and causing the landscape itself to disappear.

The earth became conceptually solid only after many generations of surface-forming rites had been practiced and set in place. The stringent dictates of the metaformic rites involved great discipline of mind and control of instinctive impulses. Not to scratch or even touch one's head or body for three months at a time; to sit in a cramped position, never to lie down, or to be made to lie down, for weeks on end; to be enclosed in solitary confinement without light or easy access to water and food—our modern culture uses these rites as punishment, torture. They are protested when used too strictly on prisoners. Yet in another context, the context of forming culture, forming human mind, extreme and religiously understood uses of separation were the method at hand. In retrospect, they were the only possible method—physical applications of the body in all its relations to the elements.

Using menstrual rite, *r'tu*, women formed analogies of their own bodies to comprehend the nature of the earth's surface. The metaphors extended to include other beings—trees, for example,—sticks were understood to be like human bones. Thus, in some seclusion rites, the woman could not break a stick or later her bones would break; she had to scratch with a scratching stick or her bones would break. She had the power to break both bones and ceremonial sticks just by exposing them to her body. In some American Indian customs, if a menstruating woman stepped over sticks, spears, arrows, or her husband's legs, they would break. Stones also became equated with bones, and the earth was comprehended as a body. The metaphors worked back and forth, strengthening each other and forming basic tools for using behavior to display thought and thus to gain some measure of external control of the environment.

Once—and this must have taken many hundreds of thousands of menstrual times during many hundreds of thousands of years—the people were able to see light, water, and earth as different elements or entities, the sky began to raise up and the world grew larger.

Lying in My Own Shade

The ancestral menstruants endured terrible disciplines to get us here; I think this every time I remember them crouched in the dark for days or weeks, maintaining the prohibition to stay completely still, to stay silent and awake, to completely control their hands and nerves no matter how cold they were, or how hot and sweaty, no matter how frightened or angry, no matter how alone. How

40

much different modern menstrual experience is, I sometimes think. We learn in school to treat menstruation as a biological event with no cultural undertones. Yet despite all my attempts to treat them as irrelevant, my own periods ruled my life.

Even though I am determined to ignore menstruation, never keeping track of or planning for my cycles, I always know when I am about to get my period, because a night or two beforehand, I dream of blood. This dream blood, vividly red, runs from the palm of my opening hand, or pools on the floor in some otherwise un-related scene, or spreads down someone's face onto their shirt. It is never menstrual blood, but the blood of a wound, of which I dream.

The cramps that always accompany my bleeding are violent and unforgettable, lasting three, four, even five days, and the first two days are completely incapacitating, so I must stay in bed, head under covers, pale and dull-eyed, in a stupor.

In the first hours after my period starts, I have a peculiar, dis-tinctive, bee-buzz feeling, a metallic taste, and a heavy in-turning lethargy that is not unpleasant. During my forties, I learn to rec-ognize this as a psychic state. It completely removes me from the busy, conscious, daily course I have been on, turns me inward where "I" do not exist. Only the menstrual state, and the pain— "it"—exists. My inner eyes study its dark walls in a dreamlike daze, and something seems to talk to me. Sometimes when I am forced out into the world during this time, I do not like to talk, I do not like to move fast, I can hardly get my foot to accelerate my car over thirty-five miles an hour, and I don't care very much what others think of me. I want to be alone, silent and unkempt.

On the first day, the sullen depression that has gripped me for a week or so eases, and I no longer feel worthless and paranoid. I feel foolishly optimistic. Sometimes I compulsively eat a big meal this first day, including salt, fat, meat, and beer.

The cramps wake me in the night and usually continue for eigh-teen hours or more if left unmedicated; seven or eight if I take pain

41

pills several at a time, swallowing a little bread with them in hopes I won't vomit them up. The cramping takes me repeatedly to the bathroom, where I clench and cry, sweat and curse, pray and make wild promises.

When the completely gripping pains pass, I begin to feel joyfully renewed and childlike. I am tired and sleep, and awake with fresh insights and perspectives, often with exact solutions to problems of both work and personal life puzzling me before my period started. Sometimes toward the end I am ecstatic, experiencing mundane reality as "freshly washed," the world renewed with colors brighter, shapes more defined, friends dearer. I come to love this sense of revitalization, zest, and vigor, though it has no social recognition, so I keep it inside, a secret power.

Chapter 3

Crossing the Great Abyss

I F   T H E human race consisted of females alone, the connection between the moon and the womb might have resulted in some insights acted out through hiding from light, covering the menstruant with brush and other elementals of the seclusion rite, but human culture would not have burst forth with the language, tools, and structures it has today. Fortunately, our ancestress had another piece of the puzzle to work with besides blood, water, and the moon; she had a mate, and sons, and as they did not menstruate, they did not have a direct connection to the moon's path and to the human comprehension of cycles. The necessity of women to teach their special knowledge, not only to their daughters, but to their sons—for whom it would always be a mystery outside themselves—and the methods the males devised to display their comprehension, are what has created human culture over the millennia.

The Great Abyss that ancestor women stepped across repeatedly to get us where we are today fills me with awe; yet the Abyss for men is even greater. For if the Abyss from animal mind to human mind was a great yawning cavern for females, for males it was infinitely broader and more mysterious. They had to find ways to comprehend and identify with ideas contained in rites that were completely based in blood cycles, physiological states their bodies did not experience. They had to understand the complete abstraction of women's menstruation before they could learn the measurements it made possible.

The men achieved this comprehension, which had to be physical, in a number of ways. While women bonded through entrainment with their common flow of blood, including birth blood, and created an increasing complex of rites, men bonded and created rites entirely their own, yet centered on exactly the same subject. Probably the most obvious and easiest crossover rite was a translation of menstruation into bloodletting. That all blood is menstrual blood is well-illustrated by practices of men in which they deliberately produce blood from their own bodies.

"Parallel menstrual rites" include boys' puberty ceremonies involving bloodletting, special instruction by their elders, imitation of menstrual taboos, and induced visionary or hallucinatory states. According to ethnographical accounts of California Indian tribes, especially of last century, boys had far fewer and less elaborate puberty rites than girls, but the male rites, though sparser, instruct us about how information crosses between the genders.

Men undertook menstrual abstractions in the most physical manner possible. They bled deliberately in formal rites whose parameters were identical, though not as elaborate, as those surrounding their sisters, mothers, and wives. Quite literally, boys and men entrained their own blood with the flow of their female relatives, weaving themselves into the metaformic web of human mind. Mythology says they also induced bleeding in women's bodies, and this, too, gave them identification with menstrual power and access to human mind. It also gave them the peculiar human quality of blood power through premeditated murder.

Male Menstruation

In the beginning the men were animals and lived alone; women lived together in the sky and were happy. Every night the women descended from the sky on a long cord, eating the food with both of their "mouths." Then one day the men threw stones at the women, knocking out their teeth so that they bled from both "mouths." This created menstruation.[1]

This story from northern Argentina suggests an ancient sacrificial rite that led to the instruction and identification of men with the sky knowledge imparted by menstruation. Because the women bled from their mouths (equated in the story with their vaginas) as a result of the men's action, the men had a direct, physical part in the blood power rite. Menstruation was then a public event, conscious to both sexes, and therefore "created" by the men.

The next logical step in creation of consciousness through identification with blood was for men to knock out a boy's tooth at puberty in order to produce a male "bleeding mouth": "Among the Australian tribes it was a common practice to knock out one or more of a boy's front teeth at those ceremonies of initiation to which every male member had to submit before he could enjoy the rights and privileges of a full grown man. . . . In some of the tribes about the river Darling, in New South Wales, the extracted tooth was placed under the bark of a tree near a river or water-hole; if the bark grew over the tooth, or if the tooth fell into the water, all was well; but if it were exposed and the ants ran over it, the natives believed that the boy would suffer from a disease of the mouth." In other cases, all the men in turn kept care of the boy's tooth, before finally passing it to the boy's father.[2]

The most extreme and the most informative parallel to menstruation is subcision. An operation on the penis that is unabashedly imitative of menstruation, subcision reshapes the penis to resemble a vulva by splitting it along its length, with the scar being periodically reopened so that blood can drip down over the man's lower body.

> The idea is that when the split penis is held upright against the man's abdomen it resembles a menstruating vagina. This extreme operation, or subcision, was reportedly done in New Guinea, Australia, the Philippines, and Africa. In some places in New Guinea, the word for the cut penis is the same as a word meaning 'the one with the vulva'; in others the blood that is periodically caused to flow from the wound is called 'man's menstruation.' Another people say that the blood flowing from the wound is no longer the man's blood:

45

Since it has been sung over and made strong, it is the same as the menstrual blood of 'the old Wawilak women' [the ancestral sister creators who first recognized the synchronization of menstrual with lochial, or birth, blood].[3]

At least some of the men's subcision rites in Australia were timed with the new moon, according to Chris Knight, meaning that men learned how to synchronize with the lunar cycle very directly by imitating menstrual synchronization with their own blood.

Circumcision is a milder form of parallel menstruation, performed by peoples who oftentimes no longer give it that connotation. In Africa in particular, circumcision is common. The Dogon, a farming people, use circumcision to parallel the pain of childbirth, as a method of balancing the experience of the sexes. They say that circumcision extracts the "female" (the round circle of skin) from the man, and that excision of the clitoris extracts the "male," from the woman.[4]

Circumcision is a family rite among Hebrews. The *bris* ceremony performed eight days after birth marks the passage of a boy into the family. Since Jewish families are matrilineal in the sense that orthodox Jewish identity passes along the female lineage, *bris* seems a method of incorporating the male baby into a female "blood" lineage.

The men of the Carajá and Javahé tribes along the Amazon River go every so often to the sandy beach along the water in order to bleed themselves. One of their number, usually a medicine man, uses a piece of hard bottle gourd embedded with sharp fish teeth as a cutting instrument. He slices long cuts across the backs of the men's thighs, so that a plentiful spurt of blood ensures a rich red stream down the backs of their legs into the sand. Then the long wound is washed in the river, and the young men rub their cuts with green-pepper pods and leaves. Scars last through life; the men say they feel much better after they have been bled. Women do not do this rite, as a rule. It is a men's ritual, and women do not attend it.[5]

46

Secret society shamans of the Miwok and other peoples of California initiated boys in a four-day puberty ritual of ordeals and instruction during the course of which the boys were made to bleed from their navels. "During initiation a young boy was tossed back and forth over the fire, treated roughly, had burning coals placed on his hands or neck, and finally was thrown out the smoke hole. He lay belly down over the hole and a small arrow was shot into his navel. He was then rolled down and his parents bathed him in cold water. At the end of the initiation period, a general feast was held in the dance house."[6]

Parallel Menstrual Taboos

Boys' rites treated the blood they were shedding with some of the same taboos as had developed in the rites of menstruation. While the initiate was being bled in some tribes, neither his body nor his blood were allowed to touch the ground: "In some Australian tribes boys who are being circumcised are laid on a platform, formed by the living bodies of the tribesmen; and when a boy's tooth is knocked out as an initiatory ceremony, he is seated on the shoulders of a man, on whose breast the blood flows and may not be wiped away."[7]

Besides the treatment of the blood, other rites of menstrual seclusion passed over to boys and men at puberty: "Restrictions and taboos like those laid on menstruant and lying-in women are imposed . . . on lads at the initiatory rites which celebrate the attainment of puberty; hence we may infer that at such times young men are supposed to be in a state like that of women in menstruation and in childbed. Thus, among the Creek Indians a lad at initiation had to abstain for twelve moons from picking his ears or scratching his head with his fingers; he had to use a small stick for these purposes."[8]

Boys of the Atsugewi in California "underwent a ceremony at puberty (when their voices changed). They were said to be having

47

. . . 'monthlies' and wore skunk-brush belts. The father or another industrious man lectured the boy, pierced his ears, whipped him with a bow string or coyote tail, and sent him on a power quest."[9]

In these very specific ways, men were incorporated into the metaformic mind. In addition to parallel menstruation, men have also practiced parallel birth, or couvade, keeping rigid taboos while women give birth, even experiencing sympathetic birth pains. Ancient Greeks thought the male ejaculation coagulated the blood in the womb in some way, causing pregnancy. The Tiwi of Melville Island, as well as other peoples, incorporated the male into creation in their belief that sexual intercourse *causes* menarche. (I am reminded, here, of the slang for penis, "prick," and also of the widespread male obsession with breaking a virgin's hymen, with much fuss about the ensuing show of blood, still a practice today, for instance, in some Middle Eastern and African villages.)

In modern materialist societies, men and boys often bond through some show of bloodletting, a fistfight, say, that ends in friendship. In parts of Germany, young men have scarring societies, using swordfights to draw blood from each other, and taking pride in the number or length of their scars.

Men and Menarche

Males also participated in menarchal ceremonies, especially in the public feast that so often followed the emergence of the menstruant from her first seclusion. Navajo men help make the round pit to bake the ceremonial cake of Kinaaldá; they bring the hot water for the mix and help pour the batter.[10] In many North American tribes, men brought deer-hoof rattles and other presents for the secluded maiden. Among the Tucuna of the Amazon River region, young unmarried men play very special roles in menarche; they have their own hut, in which they make masks, and which women cannot enter on pain of death. The masks are of spirits, especially evil spirits, spirits of particular powers detected in the forest around them. The masked men are called on by mothers to reach into the house walls to frighten younger children who might otherwise wander the dangerous forest of the Amazon basin too heedlessly; the masked figures can be said to scare them into consciousness. The men wear their masks to the public feast honoring the menstruant, who emerges from weeks of seclusion on the third day of the festival. Shortly before she does, the masked men grab the seclusion hut and shake it as part of their duties of enacting fearsome spirits. Their masks are of serpents, parrots, the winds, monkeys, and imaginative motifs. In other areas, young men are sometimes given the role of flailing the female initiates as they run a race; the harder times are, the harder the blow of the flail.[11] I remember how my older brother teased and tormented me with the cruel zeal of one long-trained for the task of keeping women and children awake and alert, as though fulfilling, without consciousness or structure, his assigned male role to shake us and rattle us.

For the male, blood was something he could acquire primarily through inflicting or enduring a wound. To become an adult, he was expected to undertake frightening, exhilarating, painful, and bloody tasks. Not that women didn't cut with flint, but cutting or piercing to draw blood was the primary method by which males entered the metaformic mind, and therefore something they came to imagine as "theirs."

Tribal people of North America said that male and female blood powers had to be kept separate because they would interfere with each other, so a menstruant did not eat with men, especially hunters, gamblers, and shamans, because it would destroy their "power."[12] Through careful separation, and through parallel menstrual rites, men as well as women had access to the metaform, and to the creative power of blood.

Change of the Word Man

In English, *man* (pronounced "mon") was the word for female and *wer* the word for male only a few centuries ago.[13] *Man* comes from Sanskrit, meaning "moon," so *man* is cognate with menstruation

49

and mind, and *wer* with virility, strength, virtue, and cleanness. *Wer* remains in the language in the word "werewolf," a particularly bloodthirsty predator in European folktales.

According to the OED, the word woman is made of two old words, *man* (moon) and *wo*, which was originally *wyfe*. This word did not mean "married female," however. From its pronunciation, "Weef," and its meaning, "maker" or "producer," it more likely meant "weaver," in the sense of "weaving the fabric of culture," or perhaps "gatherer." (A similar term is "spinster"). In sixteenth-century England, all manner of country "weefs" came to market to sell their wares and products: an ale-weef brewed and sold ale, a strawberry-weef sold her truck-farm fruits, an oyster-weef sold her sea fruits, and so on. The derogatory slang word "fishwife" remains as a fragment of the earlier usage.

To do some etymological speculation, a "weef-man" was a menstrual "moon weaver." Over the three or four centuries since this time, "weef-man" dropped its "f" and became "wee-mon," as you can still hear in some American folk accents, and then it was slurred into the more contemporary pronunciation "wimmin." "Weef" changed in pronunciation to "wife," a common progression in some English dialects. And as females became economically dependent on males in paternalist marriage, the sense of "wife" as an independent marketwoman vanished.

The male warrior tradition acquired another use of "mon," in the word "weapon." The "weap" part of the word means to seep fluids, as in the modern spelling "weep."[14] Wounds "weep" blood, brought about by the "weap-mon," the moon-human who acquires blood by cutting with a flint or other tool. "Man" was applied to both genders until the seventeenth century, and this earliest man, menstrual man, stands behind "weap" man and "weef" man alike. In the beginning was blood and the moon, with the irregular rhythm of metaform passing between them.

Chapter 4

■■■■■■■■■■■■■■■■■■■■■■■■■■■

Wilderness Metaform

T H E ancestral sisters stepped out of the dense animal matrix of primate consciousness on a bridge of creature metaforms—living beings that embodied ideas developed through seclusion rites. The menstruant's inner connection to lunar cycles pulled her mind outside itself, and she cast it onto other natural beings, entraining her blood imagery with their shapes and habits. Metaform, the middle form between menstruation and an idea, was applied to the wilderness, with certain plants, animals, and other creatures singled out to embody instructive and connective principles. Based in physical life, in earthly experience and observation, the metaforms of creatures and landscape became an external expression of thought, allowing us to externally communicate ideas of measurement, origination, and deity.

The designation of certain creatures as metaforms was sometimes based on their attraction to women's blood, as with certain predators. With other creatures, the metaphoric connection was in the suggestive qualities of their shapes: the serpent is the prime example. The entrainment of menstruation to the moon drew special attention to the crescent-shaped horns of certain animals, which in Africa, Asia, and Europe became metaforms for the new moon.

Of all the thousands of species on earth, only a few dozen became metaforms, some being very local, for example, a particular white tree sloth hunted for ceremonial reasons or a blood-red drag-

onfly featured in a creation story. Other metaformic creatures occur in myth in large areas of a single continent, particularly the
jaguar of South America, the leopard, lion, and antelope of Africa,
and the octopus of Hawaii. And some, especially the snake, the red
ant, and the animals of the wild dog family, seem to have gone
nearly everywhere humans went in their many migrations out of
the mother continent of Africa.

Women's Blood and the Wild Dogs

Why did our ancestral mother separate from others during her
bleeding? Perhaps the answer lies with one of the primary deities
of tribal peoples, found on the continents of Africa, Eurasia, and
North and South America: the wild dog family. Its members, the
jackal, coyote, wolf, fox, and ancestors of the domesticated dog are
all associated with creation, with trickery and teaching, with menstruation, and with death or other catastrophes in many cultures.

It is easy enough to imagine a material connection between wild
dogs and menstruation. In remote times of human history, jackals
and other predators, drawn to the smell of blood, must have sent
ancestral females up the nearest tall tree or into the nearest thicket,
drawing lines of special attention between the habits of predators,
the blood flow of women, and danger or death.

Once when I was living in an all-female collective, some visiting
dogs "went wild" for a few hours one afternoon while we were
out. They broke into laundry baskets and ate the crotches out of
half a dozen pairs of levis and dress pants! I had a number of feelings over this event: it was extremely funny, it was a big financial
loss, and it was eerie. That was the day I began to imagine the
hazards of being a menstruating human in the vicinity of fierce
blood-smelling predators, in those long eras before we learned to
use fire, weapons, or houses. How cautious one would need to be.
How silent. What to do? Hide, bury yourself in sand, climb a tall
tree.

As I have said earlier, many menstrual seclusion rites used a pit of some kind to bury the menstruant to her waist or neck: "Among the Uiyumkwi tribe in Red Island the girl lies at full length in a shallow trench dug in the foreshore, and sand is thrown lightly over her legs and body up to the breasts, which appear not to be covered. A rough shelter of boughs is then built over her, and thus she remains lying for a few hours."[1] Some tribes required her to stay in the pit only during the day; at night she was permitted to come out, though she had to remain in the shelter. The construction of a shelter of tree limbs or brush was typical and may have recalled the original retreat to the trees or an earlier rite that took place in a tree.[2] Menstruating women wrapped tree branches around their midsections to prevent men from seeing their blood, and some Asian and South American seclusion rites included hanging the menstruant off the ground in a hammock or suspending her in a cage several feet off the ground, perhaps in imitation of being in a tree. Folk tradition is full of fears of walking under certain trees or under ladders or under houses raised on stilts, all of which refer to men's need to be careful lest menstrual blood fall on them.[4] I wonder if children's tree houses aren't remnants of what at one time were seclusion huts located in trees, high above wild dogs.

Chris Knight theorizes that in the Pleistocene, among bands of protohumans living on the coast of East Africa, the females had periods well-synchronized, not only with each other, but with the repetitive cycle of the moon and the tides.[5] I think of this seaside band, and imagine that when wild dogs came sniffing around, the protopeople must have run up trees or into the sea. Females who had made the connection between their menstrual blood and the attention of predators, and who ran up into a tree alone while the rest gathered food, or who buried themselves and the smell of their blood in the sand, prevented the loss of members of the band. They could spend less energy running from wild dogs, more time gathering food, have less risk of babies washed away by waves. The menstruant's seclusion was thus a kind of sacrifice, for the farther the band distanced themselves from her while she bled, the safer they were. But the more the females were synchronized with each

53

other, the more likely they were to go into menstrual seclusion several at a time, with older female caretakers whose cooperation would enhance their survival as well, and their ability to find the band again.

Other predators appear in myths playing the same part as members of the wild dog family. In South and Central America, the jaguar is sometimes mythically identified as a dog and as having the same metaphoric function as the dog.[6] The Bambara people say that a creative female spirit, Muso Koroni, takes the form of a black leopard; she causes menstruation by slashing women with her claws.[7] Other great cats appear in these ancient stories, and beliefs about the domesticated cat—that it lives nine lives and has twenty-eight kittens—are also woven into menstrual mythology. The cat has a long association with the wisewoman or sorceress in European folklore and religious history. During centuries of persecution of witches, huge numbers of domestic cats were sacrificed as well.

Some menstrual taboos included dogs—the menstruant could not eat food touched by a dog or touch the dog itself. The Kogi people of Columbia specify that during her seven-day menarchal seclusion in a dark part of her parent's house, the girl may not look at a dog. Dogs are believed to have been the first domesticated animal, and hunting dogs were used by women as well as male hunters among the Tiwi people of the South Pacific and the Patagonians at the southern tip of South America, as well as in the tribes of the far north.

Members of the wild dog family are widespread over the earth, and some peoples' mythology connects them to menstruation and the teaching of primary knowledge to humans. In one Navajo creation story, the First World contained only Man, Woman, and Coyote. According to the Miwok people of North America, Coyote *created* menstruation, and it is reasonable to suppose that, quite literally, by drawing the severest attention to the women's condition, the coyote family and other wild dog species, *named* menstruation for the human family.[8]

Dogs are associated with women in many mythic traditions and firmly connected to death in Western mythology. Hecate, the Greek goddess of death, has a black dog, and the underworld is guarded by Cerebus, the three-headed dog. The folk belief that a dog's howl signals death is still prevalent in rural areas in the Northern Hemisphere. Wolves of Europe were mythic creatures of death, netherworlds, and origin: Rome was founded by a She-wolf.

The wild dog family is also connected mythically to the moon. The Moon card in the Rider Tarot deck depicts a howling black dog, and in the Medicine Tarot deck, a wolf. The bloody mouths of coyotes, wolves, and dogs after a kill and their howling during the full moon must have been noticed by our early ancestors. Coyote is a trickster god/spirit/brother in tribal traditions of hundreds of tribes of the American continent. Women in particular, treasured Coyote, continuing to emphasize his religion even after the men had moved the focus of their religious activities to Sky. For the Miwok of California, Coyote created death as well as menstruation, and for many others, he is part of a flood or other creation myth. The menstrual mind, reflected through its metaform Coyote, thus created the consciousness of death and the distinctly human approach to dying.

In Africa, the jackal was a major teaching metaform, about menstruation, death, and much more. The jackal evolved in the complexity of the ancient Egyptian pantheons into one of the greatest of the gods—Anubis, guardian of the dead and messenger of Osiris. In painting and sculpture, Anubis is represented as a tall figure with a jackal head.

The Jackal and the Red Ant Mound

According to Ogotemmêli, a philosopher of the Dogon, the jackal was the first son of the earth mother, whose vulva was the red ant mound.[9] As he mated incestuously with his mother, the jackal created menstruation. The Dogon people credit their first comprehension of death to the red ant mound, the menstruating vulva of the

55

earth. In the beginning, according to the Dogon philosopher, a person who died was carried into the underworld by the red ants, and stayed living down there. This metaform, then, posits menstrual blood as a life force similar to the vigorous, continually moving line of large red ants. And like menstrual powers of decomposition and the unraveling of consciousness, the line of ants made the dead disappear, swallowed them into the womb of mother earth. Thus, a natural event was singled out for special attention because it could be connected to menstruation and turned into a metaform, extending the mental parameters of the menstrual origin story.

It is not only in Africa that red ants are associated with menstruation. Stinging by red ants is part of a menarchal rite from South America, and in North America, women of the Kitanemuk people used red ants as a treatment for complications with menstruation or childbirth—the ants were allowed to bite the body or were swallowed. Among these desert mountain people who once lived in the Tehachapi Mountains at the southern end of the San Joaquin Valley of California, boys underwent a puberty rite that encouraged them to have visions, fasting and drinking the juice of tobacco or datura. A boy "who wished additional power could acquire it by taking ants. After a three-day fast, a boy consulted an older man, who took him to a secluded spot in the hills. The boy would lie down and the other men would drop ants into his mouth for him to ingest. The boy went into a coma for several hours. After he awoke, the old man prayed, describing what the boy had seen and referring to mythological figures."[10] One Navajo creation story says that the First World consisted only of ants. Some South American tribes use ants and bees to sting young people at puberty to make them industrious, to "wake them up." In European folklore, too, the ant is remembered as a model for industry and co-operative effort.

The Hopi credit the ant with teaching people how to live underground, and how to store food; the Dogon credit the red ant with teaching them how to build their houses above ground. Although there are hundreds of varieties of ants, it is the red ant, aggressive and venomous, that has attracted most human attention. What may initially have attracted the human eye to the red ant was the mound of its home, a line of red streaming from the opening, imagined as the earth's vagina of life and death. This image could have been used as one of the very earliest communications of menstrual knowledge—long before speech, dance, or drawing aided the task. By gesture alone, people could have pointed to the busy red ant mound as a metaform for the life and death principle of menstruation. Ogotemmêli's account says just that: the ant mound and jackal stories occurred *before* human speech began, when gesture and enactment, perhaps including the wearing of a jackal skin and skull, conveyed the menstrual meanings of early human philosophy.

The Snake Is Synchronous Menstruation

Of all the creatures used as metaform, the richest and most versatile, the most widespread over the earth, the most often described in drawing and story, perhaps the most meaning-filled for the emerging human mind, is the one we met earlier in the story of the Wawilak Sisters: Snake.

"Blood from both women was now flowing simultaneously, and it was precisely at this moment that 'the Snake' also flowed from its own womblike 'waterhole' and coiled around the Two Sisters and their child." Snake is an embodiment of women's synchronous menstruation.[11] This is expressed in myth when Snake "swallows" the menstruating women. The inside of Snake is in this way the womb of the Mother. Entire groups of women are swallowed by the Snake. The myth, among other things, articulates the moment of recognition between women that all their blood is the same, that all blood is menstrual blood. The story of the Wawilak Sisters with their Snake unites into one image both menstrual flow and lochial blood (the younger sister began her own flow when she noticed the birth blood flowing from her sister), so that all of women's natural

57

blood is synchronized with the appearance and habits of a live creature, the one creature on earth that most looks like a disembodied vagina.

Western minds have been taught to see the snake as penile, but I came to understand how it could be seen as the vagina when I kept a little milk snake (named Madame) for several years and observed how she stretched her mouth when she ate. Like the walls of the yoni in sexual intercourse or childbirth, the snake's mouth swells to giant proportions around mouse, rabbit, fish, or even (for the anaconda) whole deer. Snake in Australian mythology swallows menstruating women and is itself sometimes said to have inner pains and to be menstruating. As the collective female vagina, Snake defines and displays the metaphoric relationship between the younger sister's menstrual flow and the older sister's lochial blood.

The primal vaginal snake image extends several more steps in this complex and well-developed myth of origin. Snake lives in a particular place, a waterhole, river, lake, or other body of water. Natural bodies of water are, as I have mentioned, equated with menstrual blood, possessing the same life- and death-giving capacities. In the Australian myth, Snake emerges from the waterhole womb to consume but also to wrap protectively around the two sisters. In other myths, Snake "swallows" a woman into the water and keeps her there forever. The collective flow is both protective and dangerous: the great menstrual paradox of life and death.

The snake has been associated with menstruation through the shedding of its skin, a metamorphosis long connected to spiritual rebirth and the transformation of the soul—a lunar connection.[12] The word "shed" itself captures some of these rich associations. In verb form it means "to slough," and in noun form, "a crude shelter." *Webster's Collegiate Dictionary* traces shed to two different sources. One is Middle English *sheden*, "to separate, divide," from a Latin word meaning to cut apart or to bleed or otherwise leak fluids. Shed in the sense of crude shelter is also Middle English, from "shade"; the archaic meaning was "hut." Before the twelfth century, shed also meant "different," and it is this sense that comes through in the "shedding" of a snake's skin. Shed also once meant "a divide of land," and we still use the term in "watershed" to indicate a point of departure as well as land bounded by water courses. Thus the same word came to refer to bleeding, to separating, to a hut, to watercourses, and to a snake's recurrent renewal of its skin, a kind of subconscious lingual/menstrual configuration.

Snake's watery home is the earth's menstruation. This extremely important idea enabled humans to categorize natural phenomena, and to classify and define their origins and qualities. Snake allowed people to define cyclicity itself and apply it to all wilderness. In addition to its association with the primal waters of the earth, Rainbow Snake lives in the water of the sky. The band of the rainbow, especially its red band, is the snake in the sky, a reminder of the "blood flow" of rain from clouds. The rainbow is thus a metaform for Snake, itself a metaform for synchronized blood flow. So four kinds of fluid are now included in the metaform: menstrual blood, lochial blood, bodies of water, and rain.

Snake created the landscape, according to Australian myth. After their long sleep, "each of the many giant spirits, called Wandjina, created the topography in a local area and *then transformed into a mythical serpent* and entered a waterhole. Before leaving he left his image in the form of a cave painting with instructions that the aborigines must renovate the cave painting in order to cause the monsoons to arrive." [13] The Snake of synchroneity and consciousness made the features of the earth and enabled the menstrual power of rainmaking.

That people around the world and in the past have primarily thought of the snake as female, as the yoni, is evident from drawings and statues. The snake goddesses of prehistoric Eastern Europe unearthed by Marija Gimbutas characteristically have lips, unlike actual snakes, but very much like the vulva. A statue of a goddess from India portrays her vulva extending a foot or two in a startling serpent head with twisting neck and wide open mouth. [14]

The prominent Hawaiian goddess Haumea sometimes takes the form of a traveling vagina; she is also sometimes known as Red Eel

59

Woman. A related Maori word, *haumia*, refers both to an ogress and to ceremonial uncleanness associated with menstruation.[15] Haumea's two brothers are gods who appear in the form of a rope and an octopus—as though metaforms for the umbilical cord, "born" of Haumea, the externalized vagina.

The (umbilical) cord—as we shall see, closely associated with trees as well as women in creation stories—is also connected to snakes. Many people speak of a pregnant woman having a snake in her belly, or of giving birth to a snake. The twisting umbilical cord makes this comparison almost inescapable and this is what may first have drawn women's attention to the snake: in the Waw-ilak Sisters' myth, it is after the babe has emerged and while they are waiting for the afterbirth that the younger sister begins to bleed and Snake appears. The upper umbilicus would have still been submerged in the older sister's womb, connecting to her placenta on the inside, while the lower part twisted snakelike to the belly of the infant on the outside. It seems likely that the shape of the umbilicus helped peoples, such as the Cokwe in Africa, to imagine the life force of a pregnant woman as an ancestral spirit snake in her belly who helps the baby grow.[16]

There are several more aspects of snakes that lent themselves to menstrual imagery. From the snake's yoni-shaped, often triangular head slides a tongue that is a rippling flow, like menstrual blood. In modern folk icons of the snake made of wood, glass, rubber, and ceramic from around the world, the protruding tongue is portrayed as red, despite the fact that few, if any, real snakes have red tongues. The species of snakes that have most often been incorporated into ceremonies and used in iconographic art are those with specific traits that relate them to menstruation, death, and the moon; poisonous snakes, red snakes, hooded snakes, and fanged snakes. The fangs of a venomous snake about to strike pull forward into two unmistakable crescent moons, white and gleaming. The eggs of those snakes that lay eggs are generally stark white and as round as the full moon. In myth the snake swallows or, alternatively, lays, the world egg, the egg of the shape of being, a lunar shape. In India today as part of a three-day public Hindu festival, women sprinkle red powder on the hood of a cobra in its arched upright position. With red outer lips, liquid streaking tongue, and crescent fangs, it strikingly resembles the menstruating moon/vulva. Snake thus embodies the power of sexuality and ecstasy, terror and joy—beautiful, dangerous, and vulnerable, necessary. Snake is flow, of blood force, of energy, of sexuality, of life—and above all, of menstruation.[17]

The male body was incorporated into the Snake metaform by the coincidence of the snake's resemblance to the penis as well as the vagina. When men tell a male origin story, they call the snake "he," so Rainbow Snake, who lives in the water and devours women, is sometimes called "he," despite the fact that it is also described as having breasts and other female characteristics and is known as the Mother.[18] By calling Snake "he" and recognizing its shape as their own, men were able to include themselves in the origin story.

Among the Wanyamwesi, in what is now Tanzania, there were both men's and women's Snake societies, whose members were highly respected specialists in handling the many serpents in their environment. The male Snake societies spent much of their time catching the snakes, which included poisonous vipers and huge pythons; often the men slid their bodies into the narrow network of tunnels where the serpents lived; this dangerous activity could lead to smothering if the tunnel collapsed, not to mention the dangers of being bitten by a snake or some other creature. Initiation included inoculation with snake venom and also a rite that was surely menstrual mimicry: the initiate wrapped his waist in a six-inch belt of thorns and sat up all night in the dark, blood running down over his lower body from the wounds.[19]

Snake Is the Oldest Deity

The moment the menstruating prehuman picked up a snake and fed it or painted it with her blood, she entered human mind. When her sisters and daughters imitated her behavior, reveling (as one supposes) in their common purpose, they created distinctly human speech, based not in sound but in blood imagery. And over the millions of years of human development, as the metaform of Rainbow Snake accrued more and more patterns, it became such a heavily endowed external expression, holding in its parameters so much creative power, so much destructive power, and so much protective power, that it became what we now call a god. This kind of power attended all the metaforms discussed so far—Jackal became a god in Egypt and remained an ancestral spirit in other places; Coyote is a trickster and also a creator spirit deity for many tribes of native America; Jaguar and Snake were both deities for the Mayan, and the Aztec creator goddess is Snake; the Greek earth goddess, Gaia, was a serpent, and in Egyptian writing the glyph for "goddess" was a hooded serpent. Where I am using the word "metaform," others would have said spirit, creator, ancestral originator, god, or goddess.

Metaforms held ideas, not only related to religion, the web of cosmological understanding, but also to the ancestral people's science. By using metaformic imagery, people could describe the nature of the world around them, not as singular events but as parts of recognizable patterns, operating through cause and effect. By seeing the rainbow in the sky as the regulator of cyclical moisture, they could interact with it to help order the coming and going of rain—as some peoples in historic memory credited the menstruant, as she emerged from her seclusion, with rainmaking power. From richly layered metaforms people acquired the ability to predict, and to influence, the outcome of natural phenomena through ritual and other forms of prayer. In effect they catapulted menstrual connection outside of themselves, called it Snake, endowed it with creative/destructive powers, studied the creature's habits in relation to themselves, and used the information as ordering principles to replace much of instinct, raw emotion, and the inner reasoning peculiar to animals.

The Ronga people of Mozambique in the late nineteenth century brought food gifts and prayed for permission from Snake, the ancestral god of the forest, before cutting trees. Ancestors appear in the form of snakes to the Swazi people, among others. In Mexico the great earth goddess Coatlicue, "Lady of the Serpent Skirts," is portrayed in one well-known statue as two fanged snakes facing each other.[20]

The serpent metaform grew in size until it circled the earth's parameter as the World Snake, the Creator Mother who laid the egg of the world. It also became the many-headed Hydra and the Python of the oracular mysteries of ancient Greece. The constellations Hydra and Draco were named for the serpent, and the Milky Way itself was often identified as the tail or body of a serpentine giant.

The metaformic nature of the serpent in the Garden of Eden is clear from the gnostic Gospels, buried in the Arabian desert about 450 A.D., in which Snake is called "the Female Spiritual Principle," "the Instructor," and "the Female Instructing Principle." This power of instruction comes "into" Snake, who persuades Eve that if she eats the forbidden fruit she will not die, but rather her eyes will open and she will "come to be like the gods, recognizing evil and good. And the Female Instructing Principle was taken away from the Snake, and she left it behind, merely a thing of the earth."[21] But the knowledge imparted by Snake separated good from evil. Snake is thus a description of how menstrual consciousness taught us to recognize, recall, anticipate, and fear disease, disaster, death, and to understand that our actions have consequences.

Dragons and Dragonfire: Compound Metaforms

Elaborations of the metaform of the sacred serpent metamorphosized it into a dragon. I call these embellishments or compilations *compound metaforms*. The dragon is a menstrual serpent grown to mythic proportions, acquiring horns, sometimes depicted as crescent-shaped, and enormous and very piercing eyes. Just as the four directions came to define the parameters and geometry of the plane of the earth, the dragon grew four sturdy, earth-standing legs, though never losing the energetic form it received from its snake mother.

The flaming mouth of the dragon in all probability marks the uneasy taming of fire and its association with the earth beneath the crust. Fire boils out in raging volcanoes all over China, Japan, and the Malay Peninsula, where dragons became a primary symbol. (Some Asian countries call themselves "little dragons.") Wings sprouted on the back of the dragon, probably assimilations from the great bird metaforms. Besides earth energy and menstrual energy, the dragon has been associated with weather, or air energy, and said to possess—like the menstruant—the power of storms, especially tornadoes, hurricanes, and anything causing floods. Dragons were also believed to bring famine and drought, for example, the African cave monster who "eats the river."[22]

In China, India, and other areas in the Asian region, the compound metaform "dragon" remained a natural power to be worked with in cooperation and respect. The dragon of China—depicted in brilliant colors, especially red—became a central religious and scientific principle for the many dynasties who ruled China until the first third of the twentieth century. Among other things, the dragon came to symbolize the known world of earthly domain, under the dominion of the emperor, whose robes were embroidered with dragons of crimson and gold, standing at the four corners of his garment as they stood at the four corners of his world.[23] Telling stories about the dragon under the earth helped the Chinese develop the science of geomancy, the understanding of the spirals of magnetic energy under the earth's skin. The Mayan people also considered the energy within the earth as a dragon.

In India, women still understand menstrual cycles in terms of the "fire of the dragon," a description of the accumulation of excess energy within the body. The time between ovulation and menstruation is the most suffused with "dragonfire," and discipline (taboo) is required to control the wild energy: don't eat spicy foods, don't have sex or get overly excited, stay calm and do cool things. Menstruation then drains away the built-up energy until the next ovular cycle.

According to the Babylonian creation myth, Tiamat, "Mother of the Deep," made monster serpents "sharp of tooth, and unsparing of fang," who were filled with poison instead of blood. She made monster vipers, fierce and clothed with terror, and she "decked them with awful splendour, and made them high of stature that their aspect might inject terror and arouse horror."[24] None of the viper monsters was described in more detail than the dragon, the snake whose size and ferocity were often ascribed to Tiamat herself. In the myth the hero Marduk went to war against Tiamat.[25] Victorious, he cut her in half; he flung her tail into the sky to form the Milky Way and the constellations, heaped dirt over her great breasts to make the mountains, and pierced her eyes to make them run with the Tigris and Euphrates Rivers. Marduk, in a combined act of matricide and castration, formed the universe, the stars, sun, and moon.

This classic story of the menstrual mind passing over to men through rites of parallel menstruation, including sacrifice, has been interpreted as marking the death of female power, the overthrow of women by irrational male violence. But I read it as a necessary crossover of blood power, an assimilation of the male to older female traditions. Around the world, the ancient blood forms became ogres and monsters as they were replaced by more objectified understandings of the fundamentals. Marduk—a name for the planet Jupiter—perhaps stood for a new level of male warrior/scientist. He was able to set the universe in place as a direct result of the accumulated acts of "cutting Tiamat." The sacrifice/castration of the creator Mother could have been represented by the ritual killing of a designated female, by a priestess overseeing ceremonies in which a penis was ritually cut or a living snake chopped in half, or perhaps by a yearly skirmish between warriors in the river—all such acts of *r'tu* taught the same principles, passing blood knowledge from the female to the male realm.

Long before Eve's Snake fell on the ground a simple creature again, no longer a metaform, it had contributed everything to human envisioning of synchroneity and of "the World." And the underground habits of the snake, as well as of the red ant, must also have contributed to human envisioning of "the underworld." As the earth formed on the human mental plane, it acquired a rocky surface and an underworld, imagined not only as a place of death, but as a womb, entered through a vulva of some kind—a snake tunnel, an ant mound, a cave or chasm. For many millennia the map of earth imagined by human beings consisted of a canopy of sky, either solid or made of water, a strip of earth that floated in an eternal sea, and beneath the earth, the womb of creation and death.

The Menstrual World Tree

Perhaps because menstruating women sought high trees for safety from predators drawn by the smell of blood, trees are connected to women, to the development of consciousness, and to menstruation.[26] Along the Amazon River, the Tucuna people hold a celebration timed for the emergence of menstruants from a seclusion of several weeks. People dress as spirits for this occasion, one of the highlights of which is the appearance of a man dressed as a tree, whose presence blesses the proceedings. Yet Tree is also seen as the enemy of the girls, who do not attain womanhood until they throw a fiery stick at a nearby tree. In this case, it seems Tree is knowledge of evil spirits, from which the young women must consciously protect themselves.[27]

The association of creation and trees is also a strong thread of thought in world mythology. The Maasai people say they were created by a tree; many recent goddesses have been trees, including the Hebrew goddess Asherah. Helen was worshiped as a tree on the Greek island of Rhodes into the nineteenth century. Yggdrasil, World Ash, is goddess of the underworld in Scandinavia.

In the forest of the primeval era, having recognized and established through seclusion rites the difference between light and dark, women followed the light up into the trees, where, I am sure, they thought it lived, sparkling and moving in the leaves. There our ancestress made another discovery: The light was gathered into a single form, the moon (the protomoon), and it lived above the top of the trees. The moment she perceived that reality, the sky began to lift away from the earth. The women, in their mental development, began to "live" in the sky, and the sky to exist as a place in human consciousness.

Women used animal metaforms to help teach the idea of the moon as a separate entity, either white birds or tree climbers with round backs, like opossum or porcupine. Some people specify that in their stories opossum is, because of its shape, a half moon. In the following Arapahoe story, it is the porcupine who helps the woman reach the sky:

> When porcupine had reached the top of the tree the woman was still climbing, although the cottonwood was dangerous and the branches were waving to and fro; but as she approached the top and was about to lay hands upon the porcupine, the tree suddenly lengthened, when the porcupine resumed his climbing. Looking down, she saw her friends looking up at her, and beckoning her to come down; but having passed under the influence of the porcupine and fearful for the great distance between herself and the ground, she continued to climb, until she became the merest speck to those looking up from below, and with the porcupine she finally reached the sky.[28]

Cords and strings often appear in stories of women and trees. The woman who reaches the sky nearly always returns by means of a rope or cord. The original physical cord is of course the umbilicus, and all aspects of human fertility are connected specifically to Tree. Women returned to the seat of their comprehension of the moon with prayers and fetishes, ribbons and cords, candles and incantations, imploring specific things about childbirth: gender of the child, time of delivery, special qualities of the child. To protect

67

their children they hung their umbilical cords in significant trees or buried them underneath the branches.[29] This helped establish our understanding of place, home.

Wilderness metaforms must have developed the human mind through its first several million years, and in the absence of speech, fire, and most of the handicrafts we think of as our culture. Wilderness peoples remain tightly interconnected with the animal minds around them and think of other creatures as having culture too, as they certainly do, if we acknowledge the inner mind. By making metaphoric connections, the ancestral peoples made certain creatures into aspects of the externalized human mind. In this way, they were able to teach each other certain ideas about controlling their own behavior and comprehending the nature of the world around them.

But none of this explains the mystery of the box of cosmetics as my mind's eye still recalls it, balanced on my father's outstretched hand, his expression hurt and tender; my mother's puzzled face just over his shoulder. What was in that box that could possibly have had the measurement tools, the access to intelligence, to science and the world, that I wanted so fiercely? And that I thought I could attain only by rejecting it?

For some answers we go to the next set of metaforms that make up the menstrual mind—those based in manipulations of our own bodies into living expressions of ideas and world organizational principles: *cosmetikos.*

Chapter 5

How Menstruation Fashioned the Human Body

C
*lick. Click. Click. Click. Dark Chicago evening in 1946.
I am six and at the window listening to the shoes of passersby, waiting for the distinctive click of my sister's high
heels on the sidewalk. Why does she wear such strange tall shoes?
No one can answer, just as they cannot say why she puts bright red
paint from a tube on her lips and black and lavender colors around
her eyes. No one can explain why it takes my brother ten minutes
to get dressed while it takes my sister an hour and a half. She must
wash and roll her hair, then brush and pin it. She must pluck out
some of her eyebrows, shave her legs and underarms. She must
bathe and powder, and apply lotions and creams, greases and colors. Her nails must be shaped and sharp and painted very red.
Then selection of a dress, this one or that one depending on her
feelings and the occasion and the season and the time of day. Then
her legs must be encased in stockings, the new sheer nylon ones
that are so different from my mother's photos of her own legs in
thick cotton stockings, white or black. Then come bracelets, earrings, a string of imitation pearls. Then the strange tall heels,
gloves, a hat with a wide brim in summer, no brim in winter, a tiny
veil on Sundays.*

*My father and brother make fun of how long it takes her to do
all this, how much of her salary she spends on it. But she doesn't
care! She does what all her girlfriends do. She does it, my mother
says, because she's a woman. But why does she do these particular*

things, over and over, so carefully? Why would women decide to do all this elaborate dressing, while our primate cousins do none of it? Perhaps because, my father says, we have no fur and need to keep warm. But my sister wears thin high heels and sheer stockings in the Chicago winter, and so his answer, acquired in a roundabout way from Darwin, is shaky. It doesn't address the specifics, the strangeness of the rituals themselves, which I know baffle him as well.

The ancestress has answers. Crouched in seclusion from the wolf or jackal, she contemplates the sticky red blood that is the cause of her dilemma. She comes to understand that she is both vulnerable and dangerous. She fashions her body, and in the process, she fashions the course of human life.

Seclusion Rites and Body Language

A woman's relation to her whole body was regulated by menstrual law in the seclusion rites—her relationships to sex, to food, to how she held her body, how she slept, how she sat, how she walked, how she kept her skin and hair, and what she might or might not touch. At the end of seclusion, which for menarche often ended at first light, the menstruant was frequently carried, by a group of women of her family, to water. In the river, lake, or stream, she was washed. Then her hair was meticulously cared for, washed and oiled, combed and braided, dyed and decorated. Her whole body was painted and bedecked with all the finery her family could afford and that her culture found meaningful. Then, a creature of more dazzling display than any other human in the tribe's experience, she emerged from "the shade" into public celebration—dancing and feasting. At some time after these rites of body, in some cases hours and in others years, she married and took her adult position.

"Cosmetic" is related to "cosmos," entire ordered reality, and both are related to the Greek word *cosmetikos*, ordering of the world. Of other related terms, "cosmology" refers to astronomical study of space-time relationships, and also to a branch of world-describing metaphysics. "Cosmogony" means a description of the origin of the universe, and "cosmography" means a (written) description of the order of nature. These are definitions that apply very nicely to narrative metaform, human culture after writing and storytelling have developed. But origin mythology specifies times before speech, before drawing and writing, theater or song. To get back that far, I want to use *cosmetikos* to refer to the use of body arts to enact a world origin story or cosmogony.

In the course of their rites, women took complete charge of the body, shaping it, carving it, decorating it, restraining it, and displaying it with conscious intent to express and instruct in the principles of cosmogony. The body arts are thus metaforms, enactments and physical embodiments of ideas that developed through perception of the connection of menstruation to outside events both terrible and wonderful, and to the lunar cycle and other natural phenomena. The cosmeticians were originally the menstruant's mother, grandmother, aunts, and sisters, joined later by her brothers and husband. From the beginning the cosmeticians who decorated her for her emergence from seclusion were expressing an ordering of the world; they were, literally, fashioning it.

Their fashioning of themselves was a way of telling what they knew. As the Dogon people say it, "a woman without adornment is speechless." The adornment itself is speech.[1] Not only the adornment, but the flesh itself speaks, for a decorated woman's body is not just that of a shaved animal in earrings. Her stance and gesture, her shape and manner, her inner controls and releases are all reflections of the time spent in her various seclusions and beautification rites of emergence, with their special meanings of human safety, origination, and attraction.

The body arts of *cosmetikos* continued the principle of creation through separation. The earliest separations involved the removal of the menstruant's physical person from the general population during menstruation. She was shut "away" from everyday life, in

73

the bush, the forest, in the darkest part of the dwellings. Her body became the focus of intense scrutiny from the time that she began to comprehend its measurement and to instruct others in its dimensions. Her body was dangerous and powerful, so that everyone had to know where she was during her dangerous time. The men must not look at her in her numinous phase, lest they die, and lest Chaos close around human consciousness. They must have been keenly aware at all times that she was in seclusion. Warned sharply away from certain areas by their mothers and sisters, the men learned to be ever-vigilant in the presence of the woman. To watch her, and to watch out for her.

Emphasis was put on the power of her eyes: she must not see light, men, bodies of water, or in many cases, anything at all for a specified period of time. She must keep her head lowered and use her gaze carefully, strategically, for she had the eye of death as well as of life. Emphasis was put on her mouth; by extension it represented her bleeding vagina, as indeed did all the openings of her body. Emphasis was put on all moisture from her body. Not only the various bloods, but milk, tears, mucus and spit, urine and vulva fluids became endowed with special powers. Emphasis was put on her skin, hair, and body hair, analogous to the surface of the earth with its trees, bushy plants, and flowing streams.

Emphasis was put on her hands, too dangerous at times to touch anything at all, yet entrusted with the newborn and with the gathering and preparation of most of the food eaten by her family. Emphasis was put on her feet, that they not touch the fragile earth inappropriately. And emphasis was put on her breasts and pelvis, for after her taboos were used to repel possible mates, to turn their faces from her, she had to entice male attention back to her person in order to engage with them. She had to ensure their safety in approaching her. She was completely repellent one day and completely attractive the next; she was paradox itself.

The motives for body decoration and reshaping, then, have at base been religious, from re-ligio, re-binding, re-connection.

74

Women needed to reconnect with men and children. Their decorations expressed human connections to each other, as well as to the world outside the human body. Moreover, decoration expressed the gradually increasing abilities, brought about by menstrual use of metaform, of prediction and memory.

Cosmetics: Blood Signals and Paint

Cosmetikos began as simple signals of warning and instruction, enabling women to control how they were seen, whether they were avoided or approached. The woman didn't need to display her vulva, she could paint her mouth with menstrual blood—and in doing so she created body painting. Plain menstrual blood is still used as a signal in India, where "the condition of a menstruating woman is indicated by her wearing round her neck a handkerchief stained with menstrual blood."[2]

The teaching of menstrual principles to the men and the use of blood as a signal or sign of status was heightened by the use of slashing, with a thorn, flint, or fingernail. The women could create blood at will, through cutting. Australian tribal women danced during menstruation, and in a myth they cut their breasts, as if reveling in blood powers.[3] The sight of blood on another woman's thigh could start a woman bleeding, so slashing, for some people, perhaps was a method of synchrony. Women found that they could have menstrual signals visible on their faces and other parts of their bodies even when they were not in the dangerous state of menstruation. Cuts around the mouth and other parts of the face or body displayed the ideas of menstrual blood and of the "wet" vulva. Through the act of cutting, women recreated the creative power, bringing warnings, protection, repellence, attraction, and religious signification. The blood signals marked the young menstruant as having passed into the station of a fertile, fully powerful, and world-forming woman.

The mouth was made into a parallel signal for vulva by coloring and marking it to look as though it was bleeding. Lips have been emphasized in many parts of the world by lip tattoos, a thin line drawn with a thorn or flint around the outside or directly on the lips and rubbed with pigment. One rite in particular, the permanent marking of the chin with vertical lines, was practiced on girls at menarche in diverse regions of the world. The chin tattoo is very suggestive of a bleeding mouth and avoids having to make the slash repeatedly to signal menstruation. Chin tattooing typically was done with three vertical lines that ran from the lower lip to the bottom of the chin, two at the corners of the mouth and one in the center. These were usually straight lines, though sometimes they were zigzag or a line of dots.

The reason given for menarchal chin tattoos of Karoks and others was "so she won't look like a man." Among native tribes of the West Coast, chin tattooing was primarily a mark of the female status achieved at menarche. Though men were often also tattooed on the face, including three lines on the chin, usually their tattoos were more generalized. Among the Maori, for instance, men were tattooed all over the face while women retained the specific vertical lines on the chin and outlining the lips. Among some people, tattooed lines continued down the neck onto the breasts or stomach. Blood overflowing from the mouth would follow a similar course, and chin tattoos were sometimes called "dribble lines."

After learning to use the original substance of blood as a signal, women used the principle of metaform to replace blood with other red substances. They especially used the iron-rich powder ocher and red clays, though any reddish substance that could make a red dye seems to have caught female attention. Metaformically the paint was the menstruation of the earth. In Australia, "the deposits of red ocher . . . are said by Aborigines to have been caused by the flow of blood from women's vulvas in the most ancient times which they call Alcheringa."[4] Australian, Hottentot, and Bushmen tribes evidently all associated ceremonial red paint with menstrual blood, the Australians saying the paint was "really" women's blood. Typically, the paint was red ocher mixed with grease. Then white chalk and black, blue and gold, and other pigments also came to be used as body paint. Men adapted them to their parallel menstrual rites.

Lipstick, then, may be considered the first cosmetic: "Among the Dieri and other Australian tribes, menstruating women were marked with red paint round the mouth, while among the tribes of Victoria a menstruating woman is painted red from the waist up. Among Tapuga tribes of Brazil and on the Gold Coast of Africa, she is also painted red."[5] Among the Cheyenne, at her first menstruation a girl was painted red all over her body and secluded for four days in a special little lodge.[6] In China, formerly, a woman customarily put a red mark in the middle of her forehead to signal that she was menstruating, and also as a cosmetic.[7]

Pregnancy, childbirth, and nursing were also special states designated with red paint. The Kaffir and many other tribal women painted their bodies with red ocher when they were pregnant. Pregnancy and childbirth are numinous phases of life, but it was because of the creative/decreative powers specifically accruing to women's blood that the use of red signaling during pregnancy and lactation gave women enormous powers of restraint over men and the spacing of childbearing. In some tribes, by using paint women might signal "no sex" for six or seven years at a time, while they continued nursing.[8] More usual was the period of three years used by Nigerian women of the eighteenth century, who kept their bodies smeared with red earth throughout the entire period as a public announcement that they were bearing, nursing, or weaning a child.[9]

One meaning of the blood signals was surely reassurance: "It's safe to look at me now," or "I'm old enough to bleed, but I'm not doing it right now," or "Now I'm available for sex or marriage." Among other peoples the red marks meant danger, keep away, not sexually available at this time: "Don't look at me." Mouth marking and paint was a display not only of the female power to bleed, but of a range of complex signals meaning "come here" or "stay away".

All the earliest cosmetics—menstrual blood, slashed blood, and tattoos of blue or red lines suggestive of blood on the face—must have enabled women to free themselves from some of the severest world-forming taboos. Most of the complex taboos would have remained intact in the initial major rite of menarche, but more minor ones would mark all the menstrual periods after the first. Western reporters noticed that the strict seclusions of the menstruant were being replaced in the nineteenth century by milder menstrual signals, such as a brightly colored scarf, face paint, a special apron or ring, or even a smoking pipe clenched in her teeth.[10]

Whole peoples in older times studied the color red through body use. Some completely painted their bodies red (the "Red Clay People" of the eastern United States). They tattooed themselves from head to foot (Scotland, Canada, Borneo). They plastered their hair with ocher and grease, with thick red clay (South America, Africa), or stained their teeth red (Southeast Asia, South Pacific, South America), or painted and dyed their hair, hands, and feet with henna (India, Middle East, North Africa, Europe). Even now, when menstrual rite has largely vanished, women continue to paint their cheeks and lips red to impart vitality, health, sexual desirability, and self respect.

Other Techniques of Menstrual Display

In addition to using tattoos and paint for ritual purposes, people marked their mouths and bodies with bits of special carved wood and shell. Typically these "plugs" were either slender and pinlike or round and buttonlike. They were pushed through holes punctured in the skin, ears, nose, septum, or embedded in the flesh of the menstruant. Like elaborate tattooing, the process of making a large hole in a girl's lower lip or ear might begin years before the onset of menstruation. Among the Tlingit or Kolosh Indians of Alaska, following a year of seclusion in a little hut or cage, the menstruant was given a feast "at which a slit was cut in her under lip parallel to the mouth, and a piece of wood or shell was inserted

78

to keep the aperture open"[11] The Jivaro woman of Peru and Ecuador formerly wore a long stick in her lower lip following menarche. Some South American men, those of the Karajá tribe, for example, also wore long lip pegs.[12]

In Africa, women's lip plugs developed elaborately, with round and trapezoid shapes and a variety of materials and sizes. Although their original use has been forgotten, the round lip plugs, made of reddish wood or in later days of white ivory or a shining metal, resembled a display of the full moon or the sun. Some of these plugs were disks of various sizes; others were carved balls fitted with a flat base that was inserted into the lower lip. For heavy and large plugs, some women extracted their lower incisor teeth to make room for the base. Although the stretched lips healed, the initial operations were painful and risked infection, and the weight of the ornaments must have caused enormous strain on the facial muscles. Women in East Africa stretched their lips increasingly throughout their lives, inserting grooved plates as large as six inches in diameter.

The inserted plugs, pins, and plates drew attention to the mouth. They also protected it from "evil spirits," for it was widely believed that agents causing ill health or other disasters entered the body through its openings. All the openings of the face and head were by extension vaginas in need of protection. Thus, for the Dogon people, whose culture carefully balances gender imagery, the outer ear is the male genitalia and the inner ear the female. The inner ear might be protected by having a stick run through the top of the outer ear, or by hanging distracting objects from the earlobes. In any number of tribes, a woman might wear a long aluminum "stick," like a three-inch hatpin, through the top or back of her ear, or she might have a series of rings in a line up the outer ear— all to prevent evil spirits from entering that orifice.[13]

Rings and jewels are worn in the side of the nose in cultures around the world, and particularly in India. The nose is also pierced to hold a veil for the mouth. For instance, a long loop through the septum may suspend a veil of dangling pieces that fall across the mouth.[14] Protective ornaments have also been embedded around, and between, the eyes.

Scarification was also used to adorn and protect. Dogon women display long decorative scars on their foreheads representing the fertile vulva, and these deep grooves are kept oiled so they will be "wet," a positive condition in their arid farmland. In many African tribes, *cosmetikos* consisted of a combination of embedded protective objects near the orifices and elaborate scarification using bars, dots, Vs, and other shapes pertaining to religious principles and the woman's tribe, family, and status. Her body was a writing tablet before writing, covered with information. Her breasts, abdomen, and back might be decoratively scarred as well. Sometimes smooth objects such as millet or rice were embedded all over a woman's upper body—planted in the earth of her skin—for a raised tattoo of great beauty and significance.

The meanings of *cosmetikos* evolved beyond its initial task of protecting the people from the harmful aspects of menstrual creation. On the California coast, among the Gabrielino tribe, tattooing began for girls at puberty, as we would expect. But the elaborate patterns comprised a variety of complex social meanings: "Before puberty, girls were tattooed on their foreheads and chins, while adult women had tattoos covering an area from their eyes down to their breasts. Men tattooed their foreheads with vertical and or horizontal lines."[15] These tattoos became a mark of distinct identity, defining ownership of land. "Some individuals owned real estate, and property boundaries were marked by painting a copy of the owner's personalized tattoo on trees, posts, and rocks. These marks were almost equivalent to the owner's name" and were known even to non-Gabrielinos.[16] This method of designating land is reminiscent of the boundaries established by menstrual regulations elsewhere. In old Hawaii, for example, the plot of land surrounding the menstrual hut was declared off limits to the general population. It was in this ground that the women buried their menstrual pads.[17]

Tattooing may have enabled people to memorize and reproduce the specific markings of animals and fish, as an origin myth from the Marshall Islands suggests.[18] Though the cave drawings along the California coast are mostly attributed to men, it is also known that some were created by women who had just emerged from the seclusions of menarche.[19] From the ritual drawing on human skin, begun by a mother's outlining of her daughter's lips with a thorn, our ancestors may have moved onto other surfaces to express the mysteries they were learning.

Fashioning of Body Shape

In addition to coloring and drawing on body surfaces, women consciously took charge of the shape of their whole bodies and gave them the cultural significance, the cosmological statements we call "beauty." At the conclusion of her menarchal rite, a woman's hair was carefully combed and shaped, its "flow" brought under control. The most essential metaphor of hair is liquidity, enhanced through grease and oil to make it shine. In arid areas of the world were rainfall is treasured, the apparent wetness of the hair underscored the deeply held belief that menstruants assist or control the weather, attracting water and adding to the general fertility of the world. In areas of heavy rainfall, dry-looking hair would also serve to control the sky's vagaries. Hair is plastered with mud and ocher as well as oil; it is braided, cornrowed, tied, plaited, beaded, fluffed, straightened, curled, and shaped into all manner of significant patterns. For instance, women of one Mongolian tribe wore their hair in large horn shapes held in place with metal and wood, to represent the fierce independent spirit of their herding people.

Control of the hair's wildness indicates control of menstrual flow. The coiffing of the hair, especially women's hair, symbolized the ordering of chaotic forces. This need for order has also provided a motive for depilitation (pulling out or shaving hair), which is practiced worldwide.

Women shaped their bodies according to metaformic principles.

81

Were the people nervous about famine? The menstruant emerged fattened, her mother and aunts having stuffed her for weeks with their richest foods, whether she consented or not.[20] Various peoples all around the world have for differing reasons considered fatness in women beautiful, and some took fattening to such extremes that the young women could not raise their bodies from the ground and needed help walking.[21]

Women mold their bodies for practical purposes. African women often wanted long breasts, long enough to feed babies carried on their backs during long walks; and so beginning at puberty they used "bands and ropes to compress the base of the breast and elongate it." Polynesians on the other hand admired firm breasts, and Samoan girls trained their breasts to point upward.[22] In the United States, both extremes prevail, athletic women making their breasts completely vanish, while film stars, models, and sex club dancers enlarge theirs with diet and silicone implants.

Women mold their bodies for social purposes. In materialist society, these purposes can be individual and psychological. I remember deciding, at sixteen, that I didn't want to attract sexual attention from men, so I decided to be very, very thin. I accomplished this through a diet of cigarettes, coffee, and not much food, stopping when my breasts and buttocks had virtually disappeared, and ignoring the persistent cough that kept me awake at night. Body-shaping has long been dangerous: embedded jewelry can cause infections; extreme use of bracelets, leg, neck, and arm rings can cut off circulation, even cause crippling; breast implants can leak silicone into the surrounding tissue; and diet drugs do all kinds of damage. Will we ever stop molding our appearance toward some purpose? I would argue that the motives behind *cosmetikos* are too deep-seated.

The menstruant uses *cosmetikos* to indicate how she has gone about protecting herself and her society from the dangers made conscious by menstrual synchroneity. Now that the woman has the Serpent, she understands her capacity to cause or prevent the Flood, and all her society understands that human actions have consequences. Emerging from the dark chaos of her seclusion, her metaformic paints, tattoos, scars, and embedded decorations indicate safety and allurement, group identification, order, and promise of peace and well-being. Her hard-won "beauty" embodies the cosmological understandings for all her people and ensures their survival in the unsteady, floating world. No wonder her community greeted her emergence at menarche with a joyful celebration and feast. She was *the way back,* the return from fear, danger, and decomposition, to reassurance, renewal, orderliness. They needed only to look at her to know who they were and how they were doing.

■ ■ ■ ■ ■ ■ ■ ■ ■ ■ ■ ■ ■ ■ ■ ■

Chapter 6

Cosmetikos and Women's Paraphernalia

*M*y heart is beating hard, and even though I am alone in the room I move with stealth, head turned guiltily over one shoulder. I am for the first time opening my mother's purse, and I'm doing it in order to steal from her.

My fingers scrabble past the items that don't interest me, the shiny tube of lipstick, the comb, the compact with its perfectly round mirror and pat of face powder. The tiny container of red goop with the French name: rouge. I'm aiming my finger for the pouch within a pouch, the change purse with its silver treasure that will buy me the candy bars and soda, potato chips and subsequent acne that change my status from good child to secretive American adolescent. I am completely aware of what this one act means as I finger the quarters and dimes, my feelings gathering somewhere between defiance and grief in the growing cloak of solitude.

Only one other item of my mother's interests me: her cedar chest. The red wood gleams enticingly where it rests, tucked in the closet of my parent's tiny apartment, every inch of which I have explored and exploited, except that one place, my mother's cedar chest.

What is in my mother's cedar chest? Not much that she can talk about. She calls it her "hope" chest, half-filled with folded and boxed items she saved for and from her marriage in 1926. "What things?" I ask once when I am twelve, and her face is suddenly vague, as though she has reached into the magic hat to pull out a *rabbit and realized it has escaped. Lethargically she displays some doilies crocheted by my grandmother and a linen tablecloth, never used. Her wedding pictures, simple and austerely Protestant, no brilliant gown with train and veil, just a plain whitish dress. She is fiercely protective of her cedar chest, yet oddly diffident about its contents. I lose interest, and I never open it. I keep my dolls and teddy bear on top of the chest along with the dominoes. I play in my brother's engineer boots, convert my dolls from girls to boys. I practice walking with long strides, staring straight ahead, my face clear of hair, my gaze direct and fearless. I hate my mother's small-footed scuttle, how she walks always looking down at the ground, how her hands cling to each other, how ashamed she seems.*

Now that I am fifty and my mother eighty-eight, her red cedar chest is the only furniture of hers that I value. I assume there must have been a long line of such chests with wedding gowns, crocheted and knitted items, embroidery, recipes perhaps—women's things passed along a distaff line that, increasingly, forgot the origins and greater significance of their paraphernalia.

I think of other boxes and containers connected to women: Pandora's box, releasing disease and evil upon mankind; the cornucopia of Ceres spilling forth its fruits and grains; the storehouse of Inanna, in the Euphrates valley of Sumer. What were these boxes that belong to goddesses of old? What do they signify? I remember that in slang, box means "vulva." My mother has no word for vulva.

"I hated my life," she says once, furiously, suddenly. "It's been so . . . dull, meaningless. Same thing day after day—Why? Why have I had to go through it? Am I supposed to be learning something?" Her outburst frightens me, her eyes are furious points of light.

"Just once," she says intensely, "I felt understood by someone. A woman passed me on the street, and she looked right at me. I felt then that she knew me, knew something about me and was telling me about myself." Her eyes tear into me, churn my innards. She grips my arm. I feel like the oracle at Delphi being consulted

85

two thousand years too late. "Do you know what she was trying to tell me?" I shrug, helpless. My mother's bread crumbs don't lead me anywhere in her forest, her Chaos.

"It's a mystery," she says then, relaxing her grip, again shining, almost translucent with light and love pouring through her. She is a bright young sparrow. She is the oracle now, her voice delivering a gift: "The whole thing is a mystery."

My mother is a mystery to me, her paranoia, her childlikeness, her whimsy, her indomitable will, her well-hidden violence, and her metaphysical revelations have all taught me that what women are is so different from what anything in our society has taught us to express.

I'm going to imagine that this—a story of origins, woven from my need to understand her and to mend the fabric of my own life—is what is in my cedar chest.

Cosmetikos and Women's Paraphernalia

I try to imagine not scratching my head for a year, not touching my hair or skin, not if a mosquito bite swells, not if sweat runs down, not if ants walk on me, not if lice move in. I begin to understand one reason why so many women hate, truly *hate*, bugs of any kind, shuddering when they think of them.

The institution of the scratching stick must have made menstrual seclusion much more comfortable, though comfort does not seem to have been an ancestral motive. It makes *me* more comfortable to think of the women with scratching sticks, than without them. The sticks of women in some California Indian tribes were smooth, shaped like an elongated flat diamond, with grooved straight lines dyed black or red.[1] Others were long and narrow, a forearm with curved fingers resembling a hand, a shape we easily recognize as "fork" or "rake."

The original twig the menstruant used to touch her skin in wilderness settings became symmetrical and smooth, carved and multiple-purposed. It became the varied objects of *cosmetikos—*

86

slender pins for ears or lip, long polished wooden slides and tall arched bows to hold hair in place, and to shape it into meaningful sculptures. Combs were sometimes made of fish skeletons, as well as of wood, ivory, and bone. In British Columbia, a Shuswap Indian of last century might wear her deer-bone scratcher and a comb with three points, suspended from her belt.[2] In Latin and Greek both, the word for "comb" also meant "vulva." The comb became so important to women that we are seldom without one. In former times, we were buried with them, along with containers of ochre and other cosmetics.

The Evil Eye and the Lowered Gaze

The menstruant's gaze possessed a special ability to inflict harm—the Evil Eye. The Evil Eye can cause crops to fail, food to rot, babies to fall sick. Amulets, arm bands, and all manner of charms are still worn in many regions of rural Europe, the Middle East, and North Africa, to guard against it. According to ancient texts, there was also an "Eye of Life," the bestowing of which was a blessing, recalled in such phrases as "look kindly upon" or "beneficent gaze."[3] The Evil Eye has gotten much more attention, however, especially since it was believed to be as much involuntary as voluntary, making its power that much more in need of control.

Because her gaze carried great danger to men, the menstruant often emerged from seclusion with her head bowed. She also kept her head, or at least her eyes, sometimes her entire body, covered anytime she had to walk abroad during her period. In some areas, a woman's gaze continued to carry evil potential throughout her life, and she learned to veil it, to lower her eyes—in modesty, that essential menstrual word—to glance sideways, and to surround her eyes with substances that hid or diverted her gaze, made it appear less direct.

All eye makeup veils the eye: eye shadows' colors divert attention from the pupil, and eyeliner puts the eye in shadow. Long lashes veil the eye best, and mascara is a method of thickening and lengthening the hairs to make the veil more distinct. False eyelashes lengthen the hairs still more, the aim at times being to sweep the veil completely down over the eye onto the cheek. Middle Eastern and North African women wear silver headbands whose slender metal dangles or rows of coins cover their eyes. Peoples without metallurgy wore wooden or beaded dangles to curtain their eyes. I have seen a veil of silver over one eye, on a gorgeously red-dressed Chinese doll. In the Far East, the fan was used to hide a woman's face and eyes, and holding the fan so the eyes barely showed became part of a woman's allure.

Eye makeup has also been used to protect the eye itself. Ground malachite produces green eye shadow that discourages insects; it was highly favored in ancient Egypt. Other substances have cooling or warming effects on the eyes, such as kohl, made from various medicinal substances, including camphor, which even modern studies claim can increase clairvoyance.[4] Makeup had physiological effects that enhanced female disciplines learned in long seclusions, such as heightened psychism and intensely examined dreaming. In India and parts of Asia, cosmetics turned women's allure and conscious use of sexual knowledge into the artful science of Tantrism, which also made use of substances that caused physiological changes: "cinnabar, sandalwood powder and paste, sulphur paste, rice paste, saffron, nutmeg, turmeric, arsenic, camphor, conch shell and ashes. . . . Particularly potent body makeup [was] made of crushed drugs such as datura [jimsonweed], marijuana, opium and other intoxicating substances mixed with fragrant oils and colored pigments. European witches used similar body makeup in some of their rites."[5] Belladonna ("beautiful lady") was used in eye makeup by Italian women in 1500. A drop or two greatly increased the size of the pupil, which encouraged the appearance of trance and perhaps also decreased the danger of a woman's intense gaze. Belladonna also can alter consciousness, though it is a deadly poison if used carelessly.[6] The female eye, then, was reshaped both to deflect and to draw attention, and to disguise the direct, focused gaze of the "Evil Eye." These devices of menstrual protection formed the terms for what we now consider "her beautiful eyes."

Women and Shoes

When I was a child, not only my sister's spike heels, but all women's shoes baffled me. They seemed devilishly impractical, designed with no regard for walking or running. On Sundays, if I could escape my mother's attention, I hid my black patent leather shoes in the bushes and went barefoot. I spurned slippers, high heels, wedgies, shoes with high wooden or cork soles, or with spangles, bows, bright colors. I could tolerate dull, practical shoes, but I preferred no shoes at all, despite thorns and stickers. I couldn't imagine why the human race created shoes—especially women's shoes.

The answer to my puzzle lies in the world-formation rites of menstruation. As was related in the *Golden Bough,* a Western man enticed some girls in New Ireland to leave their menstrual seclusion by offering them beads. The girls sat in cages made of broad pandanus leaves sewed together and fitted out with bamboo floors to keep them suspended above the earth. The cages were inside a room. The girls longed for the beads, but they were not allowed to put their feet on the ground. Their old woman attendant went outside to collect pieces of wood and bamboo, "which she placed on the ground, and then going to one of the girls, she helped her down and held her hand as she stepped from one piece of wood to another until she came near enough" to get the beads held out to her.[7]

The menstruant had to put her dangerous feet on some kind of platform, to keep them off the earth. Sometimes she stood or squatted on slabs of leather, or on fiber mats. From these menstrual seclusion platforms, it was only a short step to tying the slabs to the feet with vines, making portable menstrual platforms: shoes. Among the Yabim and Bukaua, when a girl at puberty is secluded for some five or six weeks in an inner part of the house "she may

89

not touch the ground with her feet; hence if she is obliged to quit the house for a short time, she is muffled up in mats and walks on two halves of a coco-nut [sic] shell, which are fastened like sandals to her feet by creeping plants."[8]

The ankh symbol of ancient Egypt, associated with the goddess Isis, may represent a sandal strap.[9] This form, a loop with a cross-piece—similar to the symbol for female—is an emblem of life, and it thus makes sense that it should also be connected to the sandal. The act of tying wood or leather to the foot to enable the men-struant to walk about on the earth may have had great religious significance. The wooden slabs she had stood upon in seclusion are now tied to her feet by a magical strap—the "umbilical cord" of the plant family. The protection of the tree accompanies her as she walks, and her walk in the shoes displays the great care she is tak-ing with her taboos, her protection of the earth, and her triumph over the forces of mental chaos. With her *cosmetikos* in place, she can take her clearly contained power out into the light of day.

There are many examples of the use of high-heeled or high-soled shoes in formal ceremonial wear. The costume of an aristocratic Chinese woman of several centuries ago included high wooden shoes that raised her entire body by about a foot. I have seen a large doll from Zaire, clearly menstrual in character, painted bright shiny red, with black hair fixed in five neat rows, black eyebrows and nipples, and black high-soled shoes that, if she were a real person, would lift her six or seven inches off the earth. High heels, then, are a display of formal female beauty, and for some peoples the higher the shoes, the more beautiful. The array of female shoes in markets and stores retains the great variety of forms and mate-rials that have descended to us from ancestral inspirations.

According to the Dogon creation myths, the first shoes were iron, because iron is the color of shade and cooling to the earth. These were too clumsy, however, so thereafter shoes were made of leather from a sacred bellows, which is also cooling.[10] Interestingly, the evil queen in the European fairytale "Snow White" also wears iron shoes; at the very end of the story, she dances in a hot fire. Red dancing shoes and silver slippers are also part of European folk-lore. In the West, the female shoe thus has sexual and mythic significance. The slipper and high heel have both been compared to the vulva, and both have been the objects of male sexual "worship" in the sense of extreme attention. The shoe entered the mythic realm, and an aura of magic follows cobblers in many old tales.

Hats, Hoods, and Gloves

Because of the widespread menstrual taboo against seeing light, early woman had to devise ways to protect the sun and moon from her gaze. Perhaps the hat was fashioned as a ritual piece of clothing that would enable the menstruant to leave her seclusion hut to ease her aching bladder and bowels. Hats also allowed her to go outside for other purposes, such as gathering herbs. She would have been an eerie figure, wandering the woods at night, silent, her body shrouded from view: "At the dusk of the evening she left the hut and wandered about all night, but she returned before the sun rose. Before she quitted the hut at nightfall to roam abroad, she painted her face and put on a mask of fir-branches, and in her hand, as she walked, she carried a basket-rattle to frighten ghosts, and guard herself from evil." [11]

Some girls wore pliant tree limbs wrapped around their heads, but many other materials and shapes came to be used. The hat, a word so similar to "hut," was often shaped like a hut and called a "hood." A young Haida woman of the Queen Charlotte Islands, at menarche and for as long as six months afterward, "was bound to wear a peculiar cloak or hood made of cedar-bark, nearly conical in shape and reaching down below the breast, but open before the face." [12] Hoods were also worn by women following childbirth on the northwest coast of New Guinea: the new mother cannot leave the house for months, and when she does "she must cover her head with a hood or mat; for if the sun were to shine upon her, it is thought that one of her male relations would die." [13] A cap with a fringe veil was worn among the Tinneh women in British Columbia

91

during their seclusion: "They wear a skull-cap made of skin to fit very tight; this is never taken off" until menarche ceases. They also "wear a strip of black paint about one inch wide across their eyes, and wear a fringe of shells, bones, etc., hanging down from their foreheads to below their eyes; and this is never taken off till the second monthly period arrives and ceases, when the nearest male relative makes a feast."[14] Besides skull caps, hats, and hoods, a menstruant might wear a mask: "Among the Lower Lillooets, the girl's mask was often made of goat-skin, covering her head, neck, shoulders and breast, and leaving only a narrow opening from the brow to the chin."[15]

The menstruant might shroud her entire body in a blanket or in a long robe and hood; or she might cover her head with a basket or a hat with long flaps.[16] In Asia hats were conical and often woven of plant fibers, and sometimes long enough to reach a woman's waist. Many Native American women daily wore caps woven of plant fibers, beautifully dyed or beaded in geometric designs. In Africa, women swathed their heads in cloth; and in the Middle East, women wore the fez, a cap made of sheep's wool, dyed red. Cloth to veil the face and upper body could be attached to the fez, along with protective jewelry.

It is evident that many motives, as well as materials, formed the hat—and all were related to menstrual rite. Women created hat designs specific to purposes: to keep from scratching, a woven cap; to keep the sun off, a wide brim; to prevent moonlight or firelight striking, a full body hood; to keep one's glance from men, material that could be drawn across the face; to protect the wearer herself, a fringed veil that distracted "evil spirits." A woman might also cover her hat with significant metaforms—all kinds and colors of veil, quills, feathers, shells, beads, and so on—to number her children, name her place of birth, her station, to identify her position as a widow or bride.

The menstruant's hands, like her head, also had to be covered. Particularly dangerous because she was so likely to touch her own blood, her hands were used to signal her state. Her palms might be painted with henna, and her nails with shiny red stain. In some seclusions, the menstruant's hands were covered with protective material. In the Roro and Mekeo districts of New Guinea, taboo demanded that a "woman who is menstruating must wrap her hands in a cloth when handling gourds"[17]. In the Tsetsaut tribe of British Columbia, a girl at puberty shielded her hands from fire and sunlight with mittens, and in the Tinneh tribe, during seclusion "she [slept] with all her clothes on, even her mittens."[18] Protective coverings of the hands must have been an intricate part of many early menstrual rites, and the association can still be seen in this recent account by a woman in Los Angeles:

> My great-grandmother's generation in Jamaica believed that sitting on the ground during menstruation would cause hemorrhoids. A woman couldn't walk barefoot during that time or she would be infertile; she must not bathe or touch water. Menstruation was a woman's thing, so the men had to keep away. When my great-grandmother bled, other women in the family rubbed special oil made from herbs on her stomach and wrapped her abdomen in a white towel. She had to lie down for the entire time, and wear white gloves.[19]

How Jackal Created the Fiber Skirt

The primary motive for dress appears to have been shame. Shame, consciousness of the consequence of one's acts, and of the volatile nature of one's body, is so closely related to menstruation that the Hebrew word for "menstrual cloth" (*bos;* in related Akkadian, *ba-as-tam*) also carries the meaning "shame" or "shameful." The Sumerian word *tes,* "fitting modesty," is the root. The more culture and cosmogony accrued to the menstrual office, the more shame also accumulated, and the more responsible the menstruant felt for terrible events, great and small. In the Garden of Eden it was the Snake of menstrual synchrony and instruction that gave Adam and

Eve the knowledge of their nakedness and caused them to take up
the covering of fitting modesty and the veil of self-control and protection. After the Snake gave them the knowledge of consequences,
the man and woman dressed their genitalia with fig leaves.

By using a navel string or vine metaform as a belt, the menstruant could hold a veil over her vulva and prevent a world-de-
forming accident, like a drop of blood accidentally spilling on the
ground. The apron, loincloth, or skirt shielded the vulva, became a
door saying, "Stop. Think." The significance of the skirt in the language of *cosmetikos* comes through in a Dogon myth, related by
their philosopher Ogotemmêli, in which a fiber skirt becomes the
first Word. The ancestor Water Spirits, the Nummo, whose lower
bodies are shaped like serpents, looked down and saw that Earth
was naked and speechless. Earth was in this shameful state because
she let her son, the jackal, mate with her (through her red ant
mound vulva). The Nummo wished the Earth to cover her shame
and gave her a skirt of plaited fiber, dyed blood red. The skirt prevented jackal from mating with her again.[20] In other words, her
skirt triggered menstrual consciousness of the harm brought by
incest. The menstrual synchrony of women, in cooperation with
men, might thus have established exogamy. The health and diver-
sity of the genetic pool could be increased by turning heterosexual
relations outward, away from the immediate family. The red fiber
skirt in Ogotemmêli's account was at one time a religious object
for public ceremonial use; as he told it, long ago the red skirt fibers
were laid across the red ant mound to dry, a public display of the
religio-sexual principles. From this central place of deified wilderness metaform, the skirt migrated to the men's tradition. Men began to wear the red fiber skirts ceremonially, and to say that they
were "being women" when they did so, joking about the connection to menstrual blood.[21]

The second Word of the Dogon was also a woman's garment; it
began as a sound and went on to be the first woven cloth skirt: The
women were talking to each other and then the men joined in, and
the sound became a helix that wound through the female body and

wrapped protectively around the womb. After the fibers were taken from the women, they made the first woven garment, a woman's loincloth that covered the body from navel to knees. For the Dogon, the woman's mouth is a weaving implement, and understood to be the source of thread. That spinning and weaving originated in the women's tradition is reflected in the Dogon *cosmetikos:* a woman wears a gold loop through her lower lip to recall the first thread, a copper stud in the center of her lower lip as the bobbin of the thread, four studs on the sides of her nose as the stakes of the loom, with its pivotal axis represented in the pendants of beads suspended from her septum. Women file their teeth because they were the first warp used to separate thread for weaving, and the ceremonial warp is associated with the ant mound.[22] The *cosmetikos* of ornament *is* speech, and as we have seen, the Dogon consider a woman who is unadorned to be speechless. A man will be more attracted to an adorned, than to an unadorned, woman, no matter what other features she has. Speech, then, in its ceremonial definition is any display that communicates shared understandings for the protection of the whole. *Word* is the manifestation of shared consciousness, *cosmetikos,* enabling women to display and men to comprehend and reflect, with their own ornamentation, what menstruation has taught them.

Like the watery red fibers of the first skirt, the many objects used to decorate ritual coverings would also have been chosen metaformically. Wide use was made of shells resembling the vulva, and of shiny wet-looking red-brown nuts, bark, and seeds resembling menstrual blood. A skirt densely sewn with red-brown piñon nuts gives the appearance of blood droplets cascading down the front of the wearer. Red woodpecker feathers were also a favored metaform on maiden's hats and dresses on the North American continent. Dress developed before cloth as the women began gathering lunar objects to themselves, and as men brought them objects with sacred meaning from a tabooed or otherwise sacred place, such as the sea, or from a nest at the top of a tall pine. Many such objects appear to have been chosen because they had lunar color, shape, and luminescence: sea shells, eggs, abalone shell, pearls, and horn. For some, perhaps many, peoples, white sea shells also indicated sacred semen.

A woman used her magical umbilical string to wear these elements around her waist, and to attach them to her daughter's body at the end of menarche, to mark her as "the moon" itself, renewed after her three-day period. The obsidian blades that had slashed blood from human flesh could now be used to shape natural forms into lunar forms, to drill round holes, to curve the edges. Before growing a single strand of cotton or having yet attained the loom, women dressed themselves in stunning and gorgeous array with fundamental metaforms gathered from the wilderness around them, helping them to categorize and name its elements.

As cloth and leather came into use, they were endowed with the attributes of female skin and acquired sacred status. Whatever became the prominent dress, the long tapering pegs of smooth wood and bone or geometric plugs that had been for uncounted generations inserted into the menstruant's flesh became the pins, buttons, hooks, and ties that held the "skin" of her clothing together. These fastenings, too, for a long time, retained the older sacred meanings in their newer practical use.[23]

Woman had been sewing her own flesh together so long, embedding long tapered pins in the tops of her ears and loops in her lips and nose; making holes in her own flesh for quills and feathers and little grooved plugs with wide ends that wouldn't slide out. She had all the shapes and most of the function; she simply had to transfer the body arts outward to the new surfaces. *Cosmetikos* gradually migrated off the body's skin and onto the parallel skins to create what we now consider "clothing." Woman stepped out of seclusion in style; she *was* style. She was the human mind, fashioned and on display.

Utensils: In the Kitchen of the Ancestress

Wrapped in her sense of poverty, I grew up imagining my mother didn't own much. She had a few dresses, sometimes very few in-

deed, and a threadbare rug under the two stuffed livingroom chairs in which she and her husband sat, each in their own, king and queen of the world's tiniest kingdom. She had maybe forty dishes in her small kitchen, if you count lemonade pitcher, the finer glasses and stack of rose-rimmed plates left of her wedding gifts, used exclusively for holiday meals. She had remnants of heavy good silverware mixed with cheap, a kettle, a couple of aluminum pots, and a more-favored stainless steel one. Her cast iron skillet fried everything from savory potatoes and onions to meats, eggs, and pancakes.

In the corner of the silverware drawer was tucked a package of paper straws, which were for me. Sipping soda through a straw was a courtship rite for my mother's generation and a must-do for adolescents of my generation. But straws were becoming a children's, not a woman's, artifact. When I left home and trained as a medical laboratory technician, I worked in the hematology lab, using straws again in the form of glass pipettes (now obsolete, I hear). These straws were calibrated for close measurements of small amounts of fluid, releasing a single drop at a time—chemical and body fluids, especially blood. But these calibrated straws were never associated with those in my mother's kitchen, rather they were credited to the imaginations of men, scientific men. And when I once suggested to my physician boss that laboratory procedures were versions of recipes, I was nearly fired on the spot.

If the generations could be traced back far enough along my mother's line, we would find ancestresses who owned far fewer dishes than she. But the number doesn't matter, only the form and function that were created in the menstrual rites—of bowls and plates, forks, spoons, straws, and the whole formality of dining and cooking, of sitting in chairs with a rug underfoot.

If the person of the emergent menstruant was draped and coiffed in growing numbers of cultural objects, inside her hut significant metaforms were also accumulating. The woman's hands during menstruation and childbirth were so dangerous because she might have blood on them. She not only could not feed others, she could not even feed herself with them. This led to ingenious and distinctly human solutions.

Because she could not touch her food with her fingers she used a long stick to maneuver food to her lips.[24] Since two sticks do a better job, after a while she began using an early version of chopsticks. In other areas of the world, the wooden stick developed teeth and became a fork. If she used a mussel shell to drink water instead of cupping it in her hands, the shell needed only a handle attached to become a spoon. Chinese ceramic soup spoons of today very much resemble the elongated boat shape of a mussel shell.

Because she could not touch food with her dangerous hands she had to develop plates, cups, and bowls, and at first these were simple wilderness items: "Among the Bribri Indians of Costa Rica a menstruous woman is regarded as unclean. The only plates she may use for her food are banana leaves, which, when she has done with them, she throws away in some sequestered spot; for were a cow to find and eat them, it would waste away. And she drinks out of a special vessel for a like reason: if any one drank out of the same cup after her, he would surely die."[25] In other areas, her food was handed to her on a piece of wood or a square of leather. She began to acquire "stuff": among the Maidu Indians of California, where menarchal seclusion lasted five days, "she had a basket, plate, and cup for her own use, and a stick with which to scratch her head."[26]

In some places, as we have seen, her plate and bowl and eating sticks were kept exclusively for her use, but in others her utensils had to be destroyed after each seclusion.[27] This meant that women would constantly be on the lookout for any object in nature that might serve as a cup or bowl to bring water to a menstrual or birthing relative. Anything that would carry water would have become highly valued. Gourds, strong leaves, hollow wood or stone, a wad of grass lined with pitch. Out of the demands of their own world-forming taboos, women would have learned to plait grasses tightly enough to make a basket waterproof.

Chair and Rug

Among the plaited objects in the menstruant's hut, one of the first may have been her rug. Since she was forbidden to touch the ground with any part of her body, leaves were spread for her, banana leaves, broad pandanus leaves, pine boughs, or bark.[28] Later the floor covering would be woven or fitted together—mats, sticks of bamboo, slats of wood. From this practice, it seems reasonable to suppose, people may have developed the habit of putting wooden floors in their houses.

During her seclusions she would have also acquired the wooden chair and stool as a matter of course, because her vulva could not touch the earth: "Among the Yabim and Bukaua, two neighbouring and kindred tribes on the coast of Northern New Guinea, a girl at puberty is secluded for some five or six weeks in an inner part of the house; but she may not sit on the floor, lest her uncleanliness should cleave to it, so a log of wood is placed for her to squat on."[29] The menstruant squatted on special materials that kept her safely raised: slabs of wood, slabs of leather, woven mats, and in clothmaking cultures, pillows. Rachel, in Genesis, sat upon a special "camel chair" seat to menstruate.[30]

The menstruant was propped up with logs or branches on three sides and underneath, to keep her contained and to keep her from lying down or from falling asleep. This form of her sitting body, outlined in wood, needed only to have its parts lashed together to become what we know as a chair. Men of course acquired the right to sit in chairs, just as they acquired clothing. My father and mother each had a designated chair, and they rarely sat anywhere else; chairs now belong to both genders. But as with all *cosmetikos,* the ideology for and the source of the form *chair* belong to the menstrual seclusion rites.

From the nakedness of the primal ancestress in her elemental hut, to the menstruant's emergence in full public ceremony at the end of her seclusion, women enacted and communicated fundamental mysteries by dressing in metaforms. The menstruant's paraphernalia piled up around her—her bowls, her straws, her mats, and her plates. They were hers alone; no one else could use them without being harmed. If she didn't break them, they had to be stored in special places, kept away from others in what would eventually become trunks, boxes, baskets, closets, cupboards—and my mother's red cedar chest. Her utensils would be carefully wrapped and cleaned, kept, like her, in the dark. She would become the one with the overflowing purse, the trunks of clothing, the hatboxes, the rolls of rugs and blankets, and the shelves of household "goods" that formed the basis, not only for family and village life, but for all technological measurement. The woman would carry her paraphernalia with her. She would become the gender who—around the world—carries the largest burdens.

Chapter 7

━━━━━━━━━━━━━━━━━━━━━━━━━━━━━━━━

Ceremony: Let's Cook!

*D*uring my mother's menopause—beginning when she is fifty-two and I am fifteen—my mother becomes "ill." Her illness is characterized by extreme anxiety and mental anguish, and by social withdrawal. For one frightening year, the worst of the two or three years of her crisis, she stays home in as complete a seclusion as she can manage. She sits in the dim living room in a rocking chair or paces the floor. She stops talking or at times combing her hair, sitting for hours with staring eyes that seem not to recognize me or my father. She emerges from her haze long enough to state her food desires so we can shop for her, but she not only has stopped cooking, she has stopped eating any meat, changing from our meat, potatoes, and gravy diet to one featuring a little hot tea, dry toast, and canned red kidney beans, which she eats unheated, a few raw vegetables, primarily carrots, and some fruits. She is on no medication and is not seen by a doctor. My father mentions that the nearest psychiatrist is forty miles away and that he does not want her committed, he is afraid they will harm her, and he just trusts she will sit there until she recovers—a man with great intuition, in an era that used lobotomy and shock treatment for depression.*

Isolated from other women and with less than ten years of schooling in the rural Midwest, my mother believed that menopause could ruin a woman's life. Indeed, when a neighbor gradu-

*ally sickened and died, my mother attributed her death to the fact
that the woman "just never recovered from her change of life."*

*All by herself (and I was no help since her illness terrified me as
well as my father, both of us believing she had lost her mind), my
mother sat in her rocking chair and gathered herself unto herself,
recovered her strength, returned to work for another decade. As I
write, in her eighty-ninth year, she still eats toast, kidney beans,
and raw carrots and still keeps house in her own apartment.*

How Cooking Took a Long Time to Learn

Especially in Europe, there has been even recently an association
between menstruating women and food preservation—vinegar
sauces, brines, wine making, and the like. The connection is expressed in a variety of taboos that have continued through folk
traditions into modern times: "The disabilities of women in a menstrual state as regards culinary operations are a matter of common
knowledge in every country of Europe, not only among the peasants, but also in the higher classes. No French woman would attempt to make a mayonnaise sauce while in that state. In England
it is well known that bacon cannot be cured by a menstruating
woman."[1] Rural people in Italy, Spain, Germany, and Holland believe that flowers and fruit trees wither when touched by a menstruating woman; this is a Jewish belief as well as Christian. A
Jewish American woman told me, "Menstruation in my culture is
not kosher, and the word for the state you are in is *traif*, meaning
unclean. You cannot go in the cemetery because it is hallowed
ground and you would pollute it; you can't touch plants, or they
will die."

In Briffault's accounts, such beliefs could be found even in the
early twentieth century: In the wine districts of Bordeaux and the
Rhine, and the Chianti district as well, "women, when menstruating, [were] strictly forbidden to approach the vats and cellars, lest
the wine should turn to vinegar." In France "they [were] excluded
from sugar refineries" lest they turn the boiling sugar black, and in

Holstein menstruating women did not make butter lest they ruin it. As late as 1878 the *British Medical Journal* reiterated that menstruating women should not rub pork with pickle-brine, "a cloud of medical witnesses" testifying to the accuracy of the belief.[2] What these avoidances mean, according to my theory of the creative principle of metaform, is that menstrual consciousness—as controlled by *tapua*—created processes of fermentation, preservation, and refining, as extensions of *r'tu*. In short, menstruation created cooking, and the substances we cherish as food were brought into human culture as metaforms.

If *r'tu* is based in blood, then ceremony, with its roots in *ceres*, cereal, and *mony*—one of those "moon" words—is based in bread. Bread is moon-cereal. Ritual takes place in seclusion and is the creative/decreative act. Ceremony takes place in public and is a display of the effects of ritual. Ceremony is the feast of what ritual provides, the display of what it has taught us. Ritual is the dark moon; ceremony is the full moon. In the ritual, the initiates are raw, naked, and bent low; at the ceremony, they are adorned, finished, and standing.[3] The menstruants emerge, are washed, combed, dressed, and set to cooking. The village arrives, the men in their spirit masks, the women with their overflowing bowls and baskets, the musicians with their flutes, rattles, and drums—and everybody celebrates. Bad spirits fade into the background. Good spirits dance.

To answer the question of why humans turned from simple gathering to farming I want to broaden the definition of cooking to include the cultivation of plants as well as the heating, mixing, and shaping of edible substances into dishes, recipes, potions, and the like. Women's root- and grub-gathering attention was drawn to certain plants for reasons of that distinctly human characteristic *r'tu*. In considering the human mind as a menstrual mind, cooking is the preparation and provision of food as metaform. To simplify a complex subject, I have described aspects of "cooking" as follows: (1) cooking by establishing taboos regarding what can be eaten and when; (2) cooking by gathering or cultivating edible

103

metaforms; (3) cooking to alter states of mind and body; (4) cooking by washing food clean of menstrual dangers and, conversely by adding menstrual dyes; (5) cooking to "purify" with fire and salt; and (6) cooking by combining sacred metaforms.

Cooking Through Establishing Taboos

Any definition of cooking surely begins with the tabooing of certain foods, since this is what brought eating under conscious external control. We cook by saying what is and what is not appropriate to eat. In menstrual seclusion, food taboos were prominent and many were consistent across a variety of cultures. The menstruant could not eat red meat or fresh fish. In North America, she could not eat salmon. She must not eat salt, fat, or grease. In India, she should not eat hot spicy foods, as they would increase her "dragon power," her menstrual influence. At times, no one in a village could eat certain things. In particular, people often made taboo those animals who had helped create their consciousness: snakes, coyotes, lizards, jaguars, bears, wolves, eagles, oppossums.

My Judeo-Christian culture does not eat insects, and while I thought this was a matter of "taste," it is explicitly stated in Leviticus 11:41 that the children of Abraham will not eat creatures that crawl on the ground; they are "abominations." Food taboos sharply distinguish culture from culture, tribe from tribe, even in close proximity. In the Philippines, I am told, one's family either eats shark or absolutely does not. Food taboos divide cultures sharply when some people keep as pets (dogs, fish, birds, pigs) what others love to eat. Some Arab peoples hate dogs, considering them dirty, and won't eat pigs; Americans won't eat dogs, considering them "family," but do eat pigs; while some Southeast Asians adopt pigs into the family as venerated ancestors and eat dogs.

Salmon was so taboo to some tribal peoples on the northwest coast of the United States that a man could not bring the fish home to his family even if they were starving. Sockeye salmon was particularly forbidden. It has the reddest flesh of any and is red on the

104

outside as well. A school of sockeye looks like blood streaming in the river. Salmon was also a sacred fish in parts of Europe, along with the speckled trout, which also has red flesh.

A myth of how one people went about reversing the taboo on salmon is contained in the story "The Origin of Salmon," related by Mamie Offield of the Karok people, who lived in the Klamath River region in northwestern California: Once two sisters declared that no one could eat salmon, but Coyote decided to change that, so he cut some red bark from an alder tree and ate it in front of them, declaring that the red bark was salmon. When they saw this, one sister said to the other, "Let's cook," and they made an opening through a wall in the stream where they had hidden the salmon, and released them.[4]

Two sisters, we know from the myth of the Wawilak Sisters, embody "synchronous menstrual flow," and therefore these figures may reflect ancient ancestors of origination. They make the red-fleshed fish taboo until the male shaman (Coyote) introduces a metaformic substitute, the red flesh of the alder tree. The story is about a change of rite, and of world-change, when a new kind of people come into being. At the end of the story, the two sisters (along with their dog) are turned into quartz, while across the river, flowing with salmon, the new kind of people are performing the Jump Dance of world renewal.

In Western mythology, the forbidden apple of conscious knowledge is a central feature of the creation story of Genesis. Fruits are particularly associated with goddess mythology; the fig and date are womb-shaped and stuffed with seeds. The pulp of the pomegranate strikingly resembles menstrual blood. The little round "Lady's apple" with its blood-red skin and moon-white flesh has a particularly evocative quality, and like the fig and date, it is connected to sexuality and pregnancy. I was taught not to eat these little "crab apples." Into recent times, barren Kara-Kirghiz women of Central Asia rolled on the ground under a solitary apple tree to gain fertility.[5]

105

In the Sumerian mythic drama "Inanna Meets the God of Wisdom," the vulva of the goddess is directly connected to the apple tree:

> She went to the sheepfold, to the shepherd.
> She leaned back against the apple tree.
> When she leaned against the apple tree, her vulva was wondrous to
>   behold.[6]

The apple tree was associated both with the star goddess Inanna and her lover/husband Dumuzi, Adamuzi, Adam—the "red clay man," who was both shepherd and bull god in the area spilling out from the Tigris-Euphrates valleys and encompassing the region of the Garden of Eden as described in Genesis. The apple Inanna/Eve offers the man is a metaform for the knowledge of differentiation (and consequent shame) accumulated through millennia of menstrual rites. The forbidding of the fruit is an act of taboo, one that trickster Snake persuades the woman to break.

We cook by specifying not only what to eat but also when it is appropriate to eat, and when not. When menarche or menstruation is over, that is the time to eat foods tabooed during seclusion. After her emergence from seclusion, the menstruant's entire community, or at least her extended family, often participated in a feast.

In my family, we eat very little on Sunday until late afternoon, when we have the largest meal of the week, always based on a celebrated roasted meat that has to be discussed and admired in detail before, during, and after cooking. My father cooks or supervises the ceremonial meals. My mother cooks the everyday food and does the shopping and meal planning. The kitchen and most of its contents are "hers." Her recipes are simple. She specializes in five or six meals handed down to her: white boiled beans served with ketchup; bacon, and eggs; liver and onions; pork chops and brown beans with mustard and molasses; deviled eggs sprinkled with paprika; creamed tuna on toast; and the world's absolutely best, most beautiful, and most irresistible cherry pie. One way my mother's food metaforms differ from my father's is in the amount of actual blood present. While my father likes his meat rare, my mother overcooks everything and then often "dresses" it in red or orange sauces.

If it was natural for the protohuman remote ancestors to eat raw vegetables, nuts and fruits, insects, eggs, and occasional rats and birds, then where did our elaborate system of food production and presentation—my mother's fancy cherry pies—come from? From the menstrual mind.

Cooking by Gathering and Growing Metaforms

Many researchers, for example, Evelyn Reed, believe that women began agriculture by expanding plant- and insect-gathering techniques through use of the digging stick.[7] The ancient females began transferring the roots they dug to other terrain, carrying them to their favored dwelling areas, and thus beginning a process of selective planting. The plants they chose for close attention were, as we shall see, those with ritual significance.

The heavy burden of farming and intensive gardening carried by women around the world reflects its origins as women's invention, with work traditions held in place through religious ideology centered in female history. In some cultures still, only women do the planting, tilling, and harvesting. It is not that men created farming and then somehow enslaved women to do most of the work for them, but rather that many women have not found methods (ideology) for shifting some of the burden to men, and men take advantage of women's self-containment. The rationale for continuing the imbalance of work often lies in a mutual belief that men won't "do it right" and the risk of crop failure isn't worth the experiment. Religious ideas separating "women's power" from "men's power" are at the root of this.

Early farming was not yet by seed; it was not heterosexual reproduction but parthenogenesis. Daughter plants grew from mothers through the splitting off and replanting of one root from the clump,

107

the whole new plant then growing up genetically identical to the original—creation through separation. In keeping with the menstrual mind, women gathered plants that resembled their ideas of r'tu, and they were attracted to red and white plants in particular. Red yams, whose flesh resembles blood, for instance, or roots such as sago or potato that are more or less white when peeled, and round, the general shape of the full moon/sun. Even bananas (plantains), which in Western markets are generally long and yellow, are most frequently found in reddish colors and in short stubby curled bunches resembling a vulva or a bloody hand (though individually, the penis).

The moon has been so important to the development of agriculture that the *Farmer's Alamanac* still uses it as the primary guide for deciding when to plant. At one time all planting was done in accordance with the lunar calendar. Onions are so closely related to the moon that they are the only crop that is planted (in the old tradition) at the dark of the moon rather than one of its fuller phases. Not only do onions have the perfect round shape and luminous color of the moon, they also put up a flower that is globular and stark white—a moon above and below the earth.

Garlic subdivides its white lunar body into distinct crescents, or cloves. Both garlic and onions were considered sacred in ancient Egypt, portrayed in murals in the hands of goddesses, and used medicinally in the female wicca tradition into recent times in Europe. Midwives in villages spewed a mouthful of onion juice over the newborn to ward off disease; medieval Europeans wore and sucked garlic cloves as a defense against the bubonic plague; and in World War Two, when penicillin was in short supply, garlic was used by the ton as a "blood purifier" to protect wounded soldiers from infection.[8]

We eat what we eat based on what the cooks have found ritually appropriate to feed us. One of the primary uses of early cultigens was for red, purple, and orange dyes—menstrual colors. Potatoes, like many other crops we think of as food, were used for purple and red dyes as well as for eating, and perhaps before they were used for eating.[9] The metaformic appeal of such crops led to fabulous variety: more than eighty kinds of potatoes grow on the mountain sides of Peru; selected by precolumbian women for millennia, yams and sweet potatoes range from huge to tiny, sweet to dry, purple and red to white.

The brilliantly colored foods of South Asia and South America represent the ancient selection of plants—cinnamon, turmeric, curry, chile, saffron, paprika, nutmeg, cloves, ginger, even potatoes—that impart a desirable red, orange, or yellow dye as well as strong sensual flavors and smells. Many of the old, traditional cooking liquids of the world are red—toasted sesame oil, soy sauce, Caribbean cooking oils. The deeper red and orange curries of food in India and Southeast Asia are colored vividly as offerings to the deities—food *cosmetikos*. In Southeast Asia, as in Japan and other places, the presentation of the food is equally important to its nutritive qualities. Its visual effect is considered part of its life-giving nourishment—because the dieties are pleased by its esthetic presentation, an esthetic based in *r'tu*.

Hot peppers, ginger, and other stinging spices were used as medicinal purifiers to chase evil spirits away, and women used tingling plant substances as purifying agents at menarche and childbirth. Gums and saps were associated with menstruation not only because of their stickiness but because they were seen specifically as "the blood" of the tree or plant: "Acacia gum, which is gathered from the African desert acacia, is also known as 'clots of menstrual blood.' It has important functions in healing and magic. Acacia itself stands for woman."[10] In America women, in particular, chew gum, and the gum is often mixed with cinnamon, peppermint or other "cleanser."

When I am eleven I do what all the girls do, I consume an amazing number of red objects: cinnamon-flavored chewing gum, strawberry ice cream and sodas, raspberry popcycles and uncooked jello, red wax that oozes sugary liquid down the chin, "red hots"—little spicy candies that dye tongue, hands, and clothing bright red—and

109

pomegranates, whose seeds drip from little girls' hands from one end of the southwestern town to which we have moved to the other. Perhaps in keeping with girls all over the world, we sought to drip redness with zestful appetites passed along the unspoken premenarchal tradition.

The association of red-fleshed foods and menstruation is articulated again and again in ritual traditions. Anthropologist Jane Goodale describes a Tiwi rite, performed by men but supervised by women, in which the men gather a small, poisonous red yam from a marsh near a sacred tree. The men coat themselves with the red flesh, and they sing songs about how "they have now been changed into women".[11]

Carrots, my mother's favored vegetable, and one she never served without praising it—"I just love carrots, don't you?"—were cultivated by her Celtic ancestresses. The word "carrot" is from the Celtic, meaning "red of color." The wild plant is distinguished from all similar varieties by having a striking red flower. The roots of wild carrots are woody and inedible, so the question arises of why the ancient women (it is a very ancient cultigen) would have brought the plant home and paid so much attention to it, eventually developing the red and orange flesh that makes the carrot such an important vegetable and livestock food today. Part of the answer is in the seeds, which were used as an *emmenogogue,* a term meaning a substance capable of bringing on menstrual bleeding. Celtic women could coordinate their collective menstruation with the seeds of plants that resembled menstrual blood enough to be named simply "reds." Parts of the plant were also useful as both orange and blue (woadlike) dyes, so carrots were used for several different aspects of *cosmetikos.*[12]

In the Scottish Highlands, women invoked fertility in special chants as they gathered carrots on Carrot Sunday, the week before Saint Michael's day (September 29). This high-spirited, sexual festival for the saint who was most closely identified with the pagan god of light, Lugh, featured the baking of a special all-grain cake (a bannock, or *struan,* used for divination), horse stealing, bare-back horseraces by both sexes, and the exchange of gifts, especially between the sexes. Women gave gifts of carrots in special linen sacks. They dug their carrots with special, three-pronged forks, and tied the bunches with red thread. The association with races, sacred light, and a cake makes this festival, discontinued in the early 1800s, a kind of yearly menarche, with carrots as the "earth's blood".[13]

The carrot plants, inedible in our terms when first cultivated, provided dye and an agent of menstrual synchrony and then were selected, watered, and encouraged to produce the big edible red roots horses love, and the varied tender sweet orange roots humans love. Carrot varieties now come in shapes from globular to penile, making them a metaform with some of the properties of Snake, and thoroughly suitable for a yearly festival of exchanges between the genders. That the red roots were equated with menstrual blood of the earth seems logical and congruent with other peoples who saw the red flesh of the yam as woman's blood.

How could I possibly not believe that when my mother went through her menopausal "mental breakdown," she returned along an ancestral line to the red kidney beans and carrots of her maternal heritage, stabilizing herself culturally as well as physically. By going deep within herself she found, even in her isolation in a male-centered world, a way back to the central feminine that worked for her.

Cooking by Altering States of Mind and Body
Cooking and herbology overlapped for much of human history; old grannies might serve spring greens or brandy as a "tonic" and put as much hot mustard on the outside of the body as in foods to be eaten. An astonishing number of plants have been used in the past to regulate menstruation, especially as emmenogogues. For example, in the ancient Greek rite of Thesmophoria, the women used the lygos vine to bring on menstruation.[14] Plants used as emmenogogues included carrot seed, as we have seen, but also sage,

111

myrrh, rue, saffron, mugwort, pennyroyal, myrtle flower, bayberry, tansy, motherwort, snakeroot, blessed thistle, parsley, and also ergot, which is a mold on corn or rye. Some plants, such as the berries of the laurel or cottonroot, were so cathartic as to be used for abortions as well as emmenogogues. Obviously, some of the plants that would bring about a menstrual flow would also serve as contraceptives. Many herbs, such as the madonna lily, were used for "general female conditions," which included such symptoms as swollen or clogged breasts, excessive bleeding at childbirth, and the like. But the synchronous timing of menstrual bleeding seems to have been a foremost purpose in the ritual use of herbs.

If menstrual ritual first directed women to cultivate or otherwise single out certain plants, by metaphoric extension they (and male shamans) found other conditions to heal with plants. For example, carrot seed was also used to treat jaundice, a condition characterized by a carrotlike complexion. By using such metaphoric affinities, herbal medicine developed, more or less effective at extending human life, and couched in terms of the metaforms of *cosmetikos*. Thus herbs gathered during a certain period of the moon were believed to hold a certain power of the moon. Witches of medieval Europe gathered herbs naked, as though to return to a primal state of ancestral power when the herbs were originally used.

Hemp, marijuana, poppy, peyote, coca leaves, chocolate, coffee, honey, datura, and tobacco are just a few of the plant products used from extremely ancient times to induce, ceremonially, altered states of mind.

Tobacco, often said to be the most sacred plant of all among Native Americans, was used primarily as a drink, then as snuff or for chewing, and finally for smoking.[15] In addition to its narcotic effects, the dark blood color must have enhanced its metaformic qualities, and the lush red-brown juice dripping down at the corners of the mouth would have been a desirable or warning look for some peoples. By using such substances metaphorically as well as physically, humans associated them with the rites of creation. The plants, like Eve's apple of knowledge, assisted in teaching.

Artists and others whose occupations require us to remain psychically "centered," tell me that it is true for them as it is for me that menstruation is accompanied by altered states of consciousness. Women used drugs for thousands of years to heighten the psychic effects of menstruation, and mind-altering substances were everywhere associated with menstrual rites, being given to girls at menarche and even more often to boys at puberty, in order to enhance their ability to have visions.[16] Dreams were believed to be given by the moon, and evidently also by menstruation. In many menarchal seclusion taboos, the menstruant was forbidden to sleep because she must not dream during this numinous time. In other menarchal seclusions, she was expected to tell her dreams. Dream interpretation became a primary office of lunar priestesses and shamans around the world, and remains a primary feature of divination and other forms of healing—including modern psychological treatments. (The visionary priestesses of ancient Greece were also associated with Snake—hence the title Pythia, "pythoness," for the divining priestess.)

Worldwide, women are recognized as the original brewers of fermented drinks from fruits, roots, leaves, bark, and grains. The brewster, or alewife, was a central figure from Africa to China, South America to northern Europe. The alewife made beer out of beer bread; she made pulque, rice wine, honey-wine, and fermented fruits of all kinds. Pineapple and many other cultigens are believed to have been used for alcoholic purposes before they were cultivated for food, and the primary use of grapes remains winemaking. Even grain may have first been cultivated for beer rather than bread. There is evidence that the fermented uses of grain preceded any other, and that beermaking preceded winemaking.[17]

Mead, an early beer, was red, as were other beers and ales, and they were used ceremonially. "Celtic kings became gods by drinking the 'red mead' dispensed by the Fairy Queen, Mab, whose name was formerly Medhbh or 'mead.' A Celtic name of this fluid was *dergflaith*, meaning either 'red ale' or 'red sovereignty.'"[18] In a Sumerian creation story, the goddess Inanna visits the god Enki, who instructs his serving man to give her beer, not just any beer, but *emmer* beer, "for my lady." Emmer wheat, an early cultigen, is red. The earliest recipes and depictions of beermaking are Sumerian and are under the auspices of a beer goddess, Ninkasi. Barley bread, probably baked twice to make it storable, may have been used primarily to ferment beer used in Sumerian taverns. Metaformic elements surface continually in the process of beermaking: the barley sprouting was guarded by dogs, and the recipe of bread, wine, and honey (possibly date honey) was a warm red color. When the beer-bread dough was mixed, aromatics were added, as though to add a "good smell" to the dense menstrual "flesh" of the barley meal. References to beer in other Sumerian texts relate it to medicine, ritual, and myth. Alewives served the beer in special public houses, and men dressed formally in long skirts drank the red liquid through long straws, perhaps a continuation of the rites of separating waters that began in the menstrual huts.[19]

In ancient Greece, grapes were so closely related to menstrual blood that they were not hung overhead, lest they drip on a person's head and cause harm; and in Europe their juice was called "blood of the grape." Claret was the traditional drink of kings and also a synonym for blood; it meant, literally, "enlightenment." The saying "The man in the moon drinks claret" connects with the idea that the wine represented lunar blood.[20]

"Lunar blood," was thus a fruit transformed by cosmetic *r'tu* into a metaform for sacred menstrual blood, available to anyone who qualified to participate in or officiate at, ceremonial rites. In mythology, alcohol became a magical drink, the elixir of immortality, the drink of prophecy and divination, the aphrodisiac of all wisdom—like the Soma drink that Laksmi gave Indra, which enabled him to set the stars in the heavens.[21] The Moon Hare of China grinds the "elixir of immortality" on a mortar and pestle, and the Scots still call whiskey the "water of life."

In culinary practice, wine is treated like a menstruant; it is kept cool and in the dark. Wine is wrapped in a towel when presented in formal dining and is served in special glasses, which, like the menstruant's utensils in the "shade," are used for nothing else and are often broken after use.

Cooking by Washing Grains: Getting the Red Out

As our ancestors gathered around them foods with the shapes and colors that embodied and extended their rituals, they took another step and began processing them. Surely one of the earliest processes was washing, begun in order to collect dyes for menstrual signaling or, conversely, to get the red out of a substance tainted by its association with menstrual blood.

Cooking by washing the red out, I would like to suggest, may be an explanation for the incorporation of grains and beans into the human diet. Cereals and legumes, now considered staples, are inedible unless soaked and heated—complex processes impossible without utensils. And as we know, the menstruants had to develop utensils because they couldn't touch anything. What motive would lead early humans to soak their food in water? Menstrual colors would provide motive, and menstrual utensils would provide method.

In a very limited experiment, I filled my kitchen with cups of reddish foods from my cupboards: red and pink beans, kidney beans, black beans, coffee, hot red peppers, dark wild rices, cloves, nutmeg, ground chili peppers, and red popcorn. (The popcorn is called "Indian Red"; it is only in modern farming that so much corn is yellow in color.) I covered them all with cold water. After a few hours, the liquid in every cup except the popcorn showed a red, purple, or yellowish red-brown color. After I boiled the popcorn for half an hour, its water turned a satisfying blood red. But I had been attempting to see if *cold*-water washing would render a red color from foods that were fundamental to the tribal societies that first cultivated foodstuffs. If women were irresistibly drawn to red, and were trying to obtain a dye, they might wash the cereals and legumes that were too hard to be eaten, or were poisonous in their original form.

The washing of certain grains and legumes would have led to

115

their softening into edibility—the wild rice and the corn were both nicely chewy after an all-night cold water soak. They were edible with cold washing alone, before the application of heat. Thus women may have "cooked" wild grains long before fire was used in human culture. Of course, sunlight would add warmth to water in the outdoors, especially if they used the bowls and cups developed in seclusion rites.

Grain is mythically and ritually associated with menstruation. In one region of Africa, where millet was first cultivated, the grain was dedicated to Muso Koroni, earth goddess of the old religion of the Bambara people. The goddess, who we have met in her leopard form, causes women to menstruate by slashing them with her claws.[12] Threshing of grain in ancient Egypt was always a sacred rite. In old Europe, the threshing sickle was frequently horn or antler, with the inside curve of the crescent lined with chipped red, black, or blue stones. The farmers in this way cut the grain dead with the crescent moon.

The connection between grain and menstrual blood comes through explicitly in a custom of the Dogon people.[23] The Dogon cultivate eight different grains. The eighth grain, the fonio, is threshed with elaborate ceremony. Yet only select persons are willing to eat it, for it is considered identical to menstruation (the two words have the same root). The grain is treated with the same disgust as menstrual blood, so only "impure" men, a special class of persons who handle the dead, will eat it. Some women refuse even to thresh it. The holy priest, or Hogon, cannot be touched, because persons touching him might accidentally have under their nails some dust of the fonio grain and thus contaminate him.

This not very nutritional grain is grown in specially designated plots. Although in Dogon society almost any sound is forbidden at night, the cutting and threshing of fonio can be done only at night. The young people of the tribe are called out to do the threshing by the sounding of a cow horn or antelope horns. They are fined if they do not attend the fonio rite.

The young men and a few strong women stand in a circle to beat

116

the grain stalks stacked on the ground. They do the flailing in a rhythm based in the number three: the flails fall in groups of three beats, with one third of the threshers coming down on each beat. The women carry the *fonio* grain away in goatskins. Sexual songs between the men and women mark the event. For the Dogon, the threshing of *fonio* is a kind of blood sacrifice, the grain falling as blood drops on the earth in payment for the blood debt acquired by the knowledge of incest (imaged in metaform as the jackal having sexual intercourse with his mother the ant mound vulva) and the whole rite enhances wellbeing of the human womb.

English folk customs recorded in the nineteenth century seem to have residues of ancient menstrual customs and their relation to breads. A number of games centered on a substance called "cocklebread," or "barley bread." In addition to its use in beermaking, perhaps at one time barley was a grain treated in a similar manner to the Dogon's *fonio* or was made into a special menarchal cake:

> Young wenches have a wanton sport, which they call moulding of Cocklebread; viz. they gett upon a Table-board, and then gather-up their knees and their coates with their hands as high as they can, and then they wabble to and fro with their Buttocks as if they were kneading of Dowgh, and say these words, viz.:—
>> My Dame is sick and gonne to bed,
>> And I'le go mowld my cockle-bread.
> In Oxfordshire the maids, when they have put themselves into the fit posture, say thus:—
>> My granny is sick, and now is dead,
>> And wee'l goe mould some cockle-bread.
>> Up with my heels and down with my head,
>> And this is the way to mould cocklebread.[24]

In West Cornwall, it was mother who called her to make "barley bread" up with her heels, and so on. Barley bread is "Cockley bread" in other districts. The terms "Dame," from "dam," and "granny is sick" refer directly to menstruation in folk language. *Dam* means "blood" in Hebrew and "mother" in other Indo-European languages.[25] "Cockles," a name for the bivalve mollusc, have vulval lips. According to *Mrs. Grieves' Herbal,* cockle is also the name for a wild plant with poisonous seeds. Perhaps in small amounts it induced menstruation and an altered state of mind, and was mixed with the barley flour.

From such examples, we can see that bread is more than "moon-cereal." Bread is "blood-cereal," and its inclusion as a cake at menarche was the weaving (or cooking) together of complex metaforms that connected the menstrual center of humanity with the plant world, seasons, light, the color red, and menstrual synchroneity.

Cooking by Purifying Meats: Getting the Blood Out

Chris Knight has suggested that using fire to dry meat and get the blood from it was part of the configuration connecting hunting with menstrual rite. Extending this idea, fire cooking thus derived from ritual "purification" of the "menstrual" meat that men brought back to the base camp. In many tribes, cooking was never done at the dark of the moon. Knight postulates a round in which half the month was "dark," with no cooking and with heavy emphasis on kinship, or blood ties; and the other half "light," centered on the full moon and on hunting, cooking, feasting, and heterosexual relations.[26]

The practice of steaming or "roasting" both menstruants and women in childbirth make it clear that fire is deeply connected to the fundamental blood metaform. Women aided the synchronization of their periods with steam baths, dancing, and massage.[27] In some South American tribes, the menstruant was wrapped in a hammock and hung over a fire to steam for long periods of time, or she might be hung near the fire hole to "fumigate." She fasted during this ordeal as well, emerging in an emaciated state, and sometimes dying of it.[28] Cooking fires were treated carefully during menstruation; in many tribes the menstruant had her own fire, which was extinguished after seclusion. In other tribes, she was not allowed to light a fire, as though its "purifying" nature would interfere with her natural flow, her power. Possibly, she was herself a threat to the vital element of fire.

118

Other substances, such as salt and vinegars, were also used to remove blood from food. Many delicious recipes in the Philippines and other parts of Asia use lime juice to "cook" seafood and other meats. The European folk beliefs prohibiting menstruating cooks from making mayonnaise, sugar, wine, bacon, and other processed foods testify to how women went about creating these recipes to begin with—as methods of "purifying" metaformic (and therefore, in menstrual logic, dangerous) substances brought into the ancestral kitchen. Because the power of menstruation is "raw" it could not be mixed with "cooked."

The making of pork sausage in rural Portugal is one such process. According to anthropologist Denise L. Lawrence, menstruating women still retain some of the older customs: they stay out of the sun, drink nothing cold, and do not eat ice cream.[29] They do not bathe or wash their hair during menses. A major event of the year is the preserving of a pig in the form of sausage, an event surrounded with taboo. A menstruating woman cannot enter the house during the procedure, lest a glance, however inadvertent, spoil the meat. Her menstrual gaze "is the means by which contamination is communicated from her body to the meat. But it is not her casual glance that is feared. Rather, it is the fixed gaze (*otho fixo*), or stare, that is believed to cause the pork to spoil."[30] Since this gaze can be accidental, her menses exerting inexorable control over her, and since no one can know when during her period this power is upon her, it is safer if all menstruating women are banned from the house during the time of sausage making.

The pork itself is treated as if it were a secluded menstruant, being covered and kept in a darkened room with the windows tightly sealed against "lunar contamination," as moonlight that fell upon the meat while it is marinating would spoil it: "Residents argue that a pig should not be killed, the meat seasoned, or sausages stuffed when the moon is changing phase lest the meat spoil."[31]

Salt was a purifying agent in the old wicca religion of Europe, and of course it is also a primary agent of food preservation, since it dries meat by drawing the blood out of the flesh. Salt was a sacred substance in many cultures and was sometimes used as money. In healing, salt was used to "draw" out illness—"purifying" living flesh of "evil"—and the mustard poultice enacted the same idea. My mother put a paste of salt on my mosquito bites to "draw out" the poison. Eating of salt was a common taboo in menstrual seclusion rites, for it, like fire, could interfere with the woman's natural flow.

Purifying techniques eliminated the volatility of the meat, which is in the blood's irresistible attraction to bacteria, mold, and insects. The ritualized practices of separating blood from meat, of separating red meat from menstruation and its parallel rites, and of using salt, spices, and fire to "purify" enabled high protein products to be kept for long periods of time. The elaborate preparation of ritual foods thus almost completely differentiated the human diet from that of the apes and the distant ancestors.

Cooking by Combining Metaforms: Bread Shaped Like the Moon

The circle is so common in our cultures, we cannot imagine not "seeing it." Nothing in nature emphasizes it—except the full moon and the sun at sunset, when its shape can be seen. As I argued earlier, ancestral people at first could not see the moon as an integrated object. They had to learn its shapes one at a time, through studying round, crescent, and half-moon metaforms, repeated through millions of lifetimes. Shaping the meal of grains and seeds into a full moon or sun shape would have been a logical ceremonial practice. Then everyone would eat the metaform together, studying the shape of wholeness.

A few breads are shaped like the crescent moon: the croissant, fortune cookies, and turnovers. Round breads appear everywhere: dark European loaves, fruit, meat, and nut pies, tarts, pizza, Navajo corn cakes, tortillas, Scandinavian and Native American pancakes, fry bread, johnnycakes, waffles, Middle Eastern pita

120

bread, Scots scones, African millet bread, Norwegian and Iraqi flat breads, East Indian chapatis, Chinese moon cakes, rice cakes, bean cakes, cookies, corn bread, rolls, bisquits, hamburger buns, sweet buns, hot-cross buns, Italian sweet buns—and my mother's cherry pie, which was red as well as round.

The rhyme that accompanied my mother's presentation of the pie, sung in her quavery, off-key voice, was "Can she bake a cherry pie, Billie Boy, Billie Boy, can she bake a cherry pie, charmin' Billie?" This courtship song implies that what makes a woman marriageable, in menarchal terms, is her ability to present an appropriate metaform of her initiation into adulthood. Apple pie, cherry pie, strawberry rhubarb pie—round shapes with metaformic red interiors, served on special occasions—a gift women present to the family, a sacred pie. (That isn't how I approached my mother's pie, however; I greedily sneaked in when no one was looking and stole cherries from under the beautifully latticed crust. And I was always caught, and chastized in such a manner as to tell me she was pleased I loved her pie so much.)

Western mythology and customs give clues that the making of round bread was at first highly ceremonial, and that it became especially vested with the royal classes and court priestesses. The word "lady" is associated with aristocracy and with disciplined, studied manners; its original meaning was "loafmaker," from Anglosaxon *laef-dig*. A Sumerian creation story begins, "In the first days, in the very first days . . . when bread was baked in the shrines . . ."[32] In the theocratic city-states of antiquity, grain was stored for redistribution in the temples. Archaeology has unearthed large ovens in early temple compounds dedicated to the goddess of the moon. Perhaps round bread, at first, was primarily eaten at ceremonies honoring the tradition of the lunar "Mother."[33]

Round cakes were also made by people who did not necessarily cultivate grain. Acorn gatherers on the California coast and other places made circular cakes of acorn meal. the women mounded sea- or riverside sand into a round well with steep walls to hold

121

the meal inside. Once the white meal was spread in this form, it exactly resembled the full moon or the setting sun. The meal was then often mixed with clay, dyeing it red. Menstrual customs among many acorn-gathering tribes forbade the menstruant to pound acorn meal.[34]

Making a cake that everyone shares is part of Kinaaldá, the Navajo menstrual ceremony. In this central ritual of Navajo life, a major part of Blessingway, the menstruant's whole family, men as well as women, participate in the making of a round corn cake, several feet in diameter, that is cooked in the ground. They use a string-and-stake compass to make the circle exact, and the men dig the hole with careful attention to symmetry. The ingredients are cornmeal, egg, oil, sweetener.[35] When finished, the cake resembles the sun, come down to earth. Like the Kinaaldá cake, the European ceremonial cake is a compilation of metaforms developed over the ages. The flour or meal is ground very finely, and only the best (freshest and most valued) ingredients are used. The European cake is often built into a mountain shape by stacking succeedingly smaller rounds upon each other; four layers are typical, though many more are not unusual. Typically the wedding cake is iced with white frosting into which are embedded metaformic emblems: pearls like the moon, roses the color of blood, and white doves.

Surely we eat our histories, our mythologies, and our moral values; we eat our security and our desires; we eat our metaformic minds and our divinities. In these traditions we maintain a slender thread of connection to our ancestral mothers, and we continue the cultural world they, and women everywhere, created.

Chapter 8

■ ■■■■■■■■■■■■■■■■■■■■■■■■ ■

Parallel Menstruations

MENSTRUAL rites, once established, gave us methods for comprehending other events—birth, illness, death, even murder—as part of the order of human life. These events were marked by their own sets of rituals, rituals that identified their essential nature as *parallel menstruations*. (I use the term here in a broad sense—one that does, however, encompass many of the individual male initiation and blood rites described in chapter 3). Menstrual cycles, then, gave human life an origin story, a shape, a philosophic meaning, and commonly understood methods of dealing with loss and illness.

Enactment of *r'tu* expanded memory and cognitive ability as it expanded the human diet and range. *R'tu* enabled the sisterly cooperation and dietary control women needed to successfully bear larger-brained babies. *R'tu* braided the mental, physical, and spiritual together in ever-expanding spirals of cultural expression. We thus led ourselves along the course of our evolution by enacting consciousness.

Birthing was certainly one part of that story, as the myth of the Wawilak Sisters shows us: the elder sister had just given birth when her younger sister began her first bleeding and Rainbow Snake emerged to wrap them together. It was their mutual blood that tied the mental knot. The prerequisite for human mind was an external reference so compelling it would catapult the mind outside of itself. The prerequisite for *cosmetikos* was ritual built around a substance considered so volatile it forced us to learn to handle it with fantastic care, and so fundamental that it defined everything of importance to us.

If birth and nursing were the center of the human mind, the same would surely be true for other primates as well, and they too would have somehow externalized their respect for nurturing and the power to bring new life into the world. Taboos all over the world indicate that in childbirth rites the point of awe and fear was women's *blood,* not the birth or baby, so that a woman who miscarried was just as feared as a woman who delivered a live child, and for that reason birth rites developed restrictions parallel to menstrual rites.[1] Menarche was sometimes elaborately attended with public celebrations when birth was barely ritualized. In places where birth was tabooed, the taboos were identical to those of menstruation: no eating meat, salt, or grease, no looking at light or touching water or food, no combing of hair, and so on. Women attended each other at this time, developing the office of midwife—literally, "middle weaver."

As the synchrony myth of the Wawilak Sisters shows, blood really began to sing to women when they recognized the metaphoric connection between menstrual blood and birth blood, as they did when the younger sister began to menstruate while looking at her elder sister giving birth, as they both waited for the afterbirth to be expelled. Blood rites in every sense created birth rites.

Death Rites and Menstruation

It has been said that women's blood was held in awe and terror because men saw that "she bled and did not die." But women bleed and do die, and men, animals—everything with blood—can bleed and not die. Death was "created" as an event in metaformic consciousness. The menstruant's entrainment with the moon's cycle of growth, fullness, descent, and renewal eventually gave us our idea of life "cycle." The moon "dies" and so do we. The moon's "death" is three days, three days was frequently the duration of

124

formal menstrual seclusion, and three is everywhere and frequently connected to death—from funeral rites that include the number three to the folk belief that three is an unlucky number to Jesus' "death" in the tomb for three days.

Menstrual rite, with its recognition of beginnings and endings, gave us many of the specifics of our mourning habits. The wild dogs, such prime actors in stories of menstruation and origins, are also connected very directly to how we deal with death. The long-ago ancestress was silent and still, hiding in her tree from predators. The silence of the menstrual hut embodied an escape from death as well as contemplation of its mysteries. Silence and stillness often accompany death rites. If menstruation gave us the external consciousness of death, we might expect funeral rites—recognition of the state of being "dead"—to be accompanied by a show of blood. And in fact, one of the most common practices of mourning has been the ritual cutting of the face and body, especially by women.

Coyote created menstruation and death for the Miwok people of California; in a dance for the dead the women wailed, wept, and danced crazily, with their hair hanging in their faces and blood coming from their mouths.[2] The Crow woman Pretty Shield described the nineteenth-century mourning practices of her people, which included slashing the arms, legs, and head until they were covered with blood:

> Ahh, how the women used to mourn! Their blood-covered faces come to me yet. They sadden me, sometimes. How often, when I was a little girl, I covered my head with a robe and cried when I heard them wailing alone on the hills. I knew, even then, that some day I should mourn, and that like them I should feel myself to be alone on the world.[3]

Ancient Sumerian texts describe a woman mourning by slashing her mouth, her eyes, and her vulva.[4]

A woman bleeding in mourning rites suggests that death was seen as a form of menstruation, an unraveling into Chaos that will

125

end with a renewal of emergence on the other side. The connection is spelled out quite clearly in the Dogon myth, which we have examined in several contexts, that identifies the red ant mound both as Earth's menstruating vulva and as the place the dead enter the underworld. Many peoples painted their dead with red ochre mixed with grease; and while some curled them into a fetal position as though anticipating their "rebirth," others placed them in resting or sitting positions that more closely resemble the posture of the secluded menstruants. A cone-shaped grave excavated in northern Yugoslavia (c. 6000 B.C.E.) contained the remains of a person who had been placed in an upright position, with lowered head, seated cross-legged on a triangle of red limestone.[5]

Mourning rites often included other elements besides bleeding that were common in menarchal rites, such as fasting, not combing the hair, veiling the face, going into seclusion for three days, wearing an arm band, sitting very still. Some peoples invoked silence taboos; some never spoke the name of the deceased again. Many of the survivors wore ragged clothing, didn't wash, and were forbidden to eat meat for as much as a year, at the end of which they were ritually bathed, dressed in new clothing, and specially fed in a public ceremony.[6] Old women were often the corpse handlers and grave diggers. Sometimes specially designated people handled the dead and were declared ritually unclean, "untouchable," exactly as if they were menstruating.

There are suggestions in rites and myths alike that humans learned the specifics of death by performing sacrifice, that we learned about death by performing collective murder (understood as sacred), often in a menstrual context. In a Tiwi menarchal ceremony an older female friend would weep and then "kill" the menstruant by striking her with a vine, which she then bound as a mourning band on the menstruant's arm. In Tiwi weddings, the new husband and male relatives of the young woman would pretend to kill her by striking her shoulders with round white feather balls.[7]

In mythology, Coyote and his relatives appear again and again

in connection with mourning. The sounds many mourners traditionally and sometimes very loudly make—wailing and sobbing—
are imitative of the howls of wild dogs. Even in modern societies,
where death rites have become more reticent, we continue to associate the howling of dogs with death and sorrow. Some peoples
beat a dog to make it howl when a member of the family died;
others killed dogs as part of mourning rites; Athapascan groups,
the Wintu, Southern Valley Yokuts, and the Gabrielino all sacrificed a dog, sometimes the deceased's own, after a death. Among
the Gabrielino the protective nature of the sacrifice is evident, for
"often dogs would be buried over the body."[8] Dogs appear in much
underworld mythology, no doubt as a direct consequence of such
ritual sacrifice. Predators first drew our attention to menstruation
and then we killed them to enact our developing ideas, as we
turned them into metaforms of death.

Illness and Menstruation

If the human comprehension of death is metaformic, our approach
to illness and healing is equally part of the menstrual mind. Shamans and other tribal healers were often women; some think originally all healers were women. Their power was great, for theirs was
a religious and a medical role. (I am reminded that the symbol for
doctoring in Western society is a staff with serpents entwined on
it—Snake again.) Healers in American tribal settings were often
"sucking doctors," curing an illness by slashing the patient with a
knife or thorn and then sucking the blood to remove the "cause"
of the illness in the form of a bone fragment or other small object.
Their medicinal bundles, besides such instruments as red and black
painted wands to direct body energies, and mortar and pestle to
grind herbs and crystals, contained obsidian blades for bloodletting.

   Bloodletting has been a common treatment for illness throughout history and in many cultures, including our own. The Dyak
sorceresses of southeastern Borneo would "sometimes slash the
body of a sick man with sharp knives in order . . . to allow the

127

demon of disease to escape through the cuts."[9] The drawing of blood was part of a great many tribal healing practices even when the person was not ill. As mentioned earlier, men on the Amazon River cut the backs of their thighs as a method of hygenic refreshment, to prevent illness. In the practices of African animism, Caribbean Yoruba, or Mexican Santería, small animals, doves, or roosters are made to bleed in order to effect a cure. Whatever its source, blood is something everywhere associated with illness and with healing.

The shamanic arts were particularly important for the spread of human culture to men, for the shamanic office could be taught across the genders. Boys were sometimes singled out as young children, and often they were boys who could identify with femaleness, who were ceremonially homosexual, or who cross-dressed or developed a separate, ungendered dress for their office.[10]

Like the menstruant, the shaman had the power of death as well as of life. Though healing and officiating at difficult births and at ceremonies, including menarche, was a major part of their work, some tribal shamans served the special office of "poisoner" and could be hired to kill someone. They were understandably held in terror and likely to be assassinated themselves.[11] In China, though ordinary women were not believed to have the "special ability to unleash the destructive power of their menstrual discharge," menstrual blood was recognized as "a powerful component of sorcerer's potions." Knowledge of its use was the province of "ritual experts, available for hire by men and women alike."[12] Though of course substances we would identify as poisonous and fatal—certain mushrooms, say, or arsenic—are part of herbal knowledge that has come down to us through the world's shamans, the poisoner's arts stem from the same source and logic as the menstrual *r'tu* itself. That is, since menstrual blood created life, consciousness, and prosperity, it also could take them away. Menstrual seclusion rite provided a concept of murder, for all the menstruant ever had to do was break her taboos in order to endanger or end the life of another. No mechanical weapon can compare with the power to kill by breaking a rule; the power to destroy a whole family or tribe simply by running down to the stream at the wrong time, by touching your head when you should not. For some peoples, the menstruant had what might be considered divine powers: she could cause flood or famine; she could make the sun vanish or the sky fall.

Illness was often blamed on the breaking of taboos. The menstrual mind wove a fragile net around human society, held in place by the specified behavior of each member, and any breach of the fabric of law caused illness.[13] "Medicine" is in fact in the word group related to "menstruation." In tribal societies, medicine is any object, substance, or action that influences spirit. That is to say, medicine adjusts the patient through its ritual use of metaform. Breaking taboo causes imbalance and, subsequently, the dark moon, illness, death, disintegration. Tribal cures—bleeding, for example—can be said to have reestablished the patient's relationship to the essential rhythms of life defined by menstruation. One does not need to argue that this was always understood in a conscious way for the associations to have been effective.

As a way to restore balance in one who was ill, many healing rituals reenacted the cycles that make us human: having the patient enter the shade, bringing him or her back into a formed world, reuniting him or her with the community. Healings imitate seclusion rites: there is bloodletting, fasting, food taboos, special washing and dressing, silent meditation, tending by family, cloistering away from others and from light, perhaps a sweat bath or sing with drumming and chanting. In a Navajo healing, the medicine man might make a pollen path from the back of the hogan to the eastern door, a path the patient follows at dawn after an all-night chant—emerging into the light exactly as a maiden does at the end of her seclusion in Kinaaldá, the menstrual rite of Blessingway.[14]

Healing amulets, like the shaman's medicine bundle, have magic in part because they have metaformic meaning. They come from creatures or other beings related to the origin story of the people, who enact its *cosmetikos* in their use. The mixture of objects is sacred and full of spirit because it derives from the logic of world-ordering metaforms. The patient is reconnected to his or her original place in the world.

Much tribal medicine has used potions or powders composed of wilderness metaforms: horn, sticky red berries, leaves from sacred trees, water from sacred ponds, bear claws, snake blood. The amulet of a Dogon woman, worn around her neck in a little leather box, contains significant wilderness metaforms—the beak of a maribou stork and hairs from a hyena or elephant tail—having magical qualities.[15] Amulets of amber (tree sap/menstruation) were also highly valued among tribal peoples.

Just as people could die from breaking menstrual taboo, they could die from finding in their houses packets containing ingredients that included menstrual blood or parallel versions of it. A poisonous packet, a *tseuheur,* used by Moroccon witches, caused great terror in the 1930s: one packet contained menstrual blood, pubic hair, newt's eyes, antimony, rusty ink, seven pebbles, seven large pod seeds, and seven fragments of mirror. The packet had been hidden in a house in order to bring about the deaths of the inhabitants.[16]

Medicine of Native Americans has included such metaformic ingredients as pebbles taken from a red ant mound, portions of snakes, powdered crescent-shaped objects, and red berries. European wisewomen and folk healers of one or two centuries ago used similar ingredients, all based in menstrual origins. It is as though all medicine began as metaforms and then expanded out to include other kinds of substances and reasonings. To the extent that the remedies suit our current metaforms, tribal uses of hundreds of local herbs for very specific ailments have passed into modern pharmacology. My point is not to say that ancient remedies based in menstrual imagery didn't "work"—obviously, they did—and this was because they were congruent with the metaformic "philosophy" of the era. (In our own era, medicine is based in materialist principles, and being metaformically congruent with our world view, the cure "works.")

Just as the keeping or breaking of taboos caused well-being or bad fortune among those who believed in them, so could the *cosmetikos* of medicine, good and bad. The potions, actions, and words of witches were feared in all tribal societies, and for the same reasons menstrual blood itself was feared, for its power over the human mind and hence over health and life. The meaning of healing is "wholeness," an idea comprehended by healers of the distant past, who guided the patient through the forces of chaos to the most sacred aspects of their shared culture. This is a complex idea, to see illness as part of a cycle leading to possible death, and to intervene with a parallel menstrual journey to the wholeness of renewal.

Much of current culture still connects menstruation to illness. The period is still called a "sickness," a "curse," though modern science struggles to free us of this obsolete idea. But at base, all our ideas and treatment of illnesses *are* menstrual. All blood is menstrual blood, including the blood we shed to heal.

Hunting and Taboo

Recent archaeological evidence from southwestern France suggests that men and women may once have lived separately and eaten totally differently, the women and children eating primarily roots and plants, the men eating primarily flesh. Although the two groups in the French site seem to have camped right next to each other, the males apparently did not share their hunting kills with the females and children.[17] The question of why Neanderthal males did not share their hunt with the women is not the only issue. Given that plants, roots, insects, and small creatures gathered by women provided a good living, why did males undertake the risk and effort of hunting, especially if the end product was not an economic contribution to the women and children of the tribe?

I would argue that men began to follow the hunt because it drew blood. In the hunt they could create complex parallel rites that enabled them to handle the dangerous substance of blood and to

131

keep pace with its world-forming capacities. The hunt gave men chances to learn the same skills of cooperation and discipline that women were developing with menstrual and birth rites. In hunting seclusions men, too, could entrain with light, sky and earth, bodies of water, and other elements of the natural world. As the nature of the hunt forced them further away from camp, human range would have expanded and the men became the ones who traveled most widely and gained knowledge of strange places. They would extend human mind far out into the world.

But while the men attached themselves to bloodier and bloodier hunts, women tabooed themselves from red meat. Like their own blood, it held the danger of drawing predators. It seems unlikely that, in the absence of fire, much red meat would be welcome to females with children. Wild dogs could be brought to a frenzy by the smell of blood and would find any weakness in the band. Once they had control of fire, hunting men and gathering women could camp near each other, and women could share meat that was "purified" by fire and roasted free of blood. Woman kept her taboos about red meat, however. Some women in North America avoided meat during pregnancy out of their very practical desire to keep the developing fetus small, to avoid complications or death in childbirth. Others in India believe that meat triggers the "dragon power" that "burns" women, a metaphor for hormonal response.

In *Blood Relations,* Chris Knight argues that menstrual taboos were instituted by women as a "sex strike" at the dark of the moon, which became menstrual seclusion. Protohuman females, he thinks, directed male attention to meat-gathering for them and their children, in exchange for guaranteed sex. Females wanted and needed meat, and harnessing powerful males to the task of sharing their kills with their mates diverted them from the more wasteful system of fighting over female sexual attention. His theory is very interesting and his work has many valuable insights, but the sole focus on the exchange of meat for sex seems far too singular and materialist. Around the world, women's cooking has shown not nearly the emphasis on meat that was true for men's—from the mammoth-hunters of Europe to the buffalo-hunting tribes on the plains of North America. Meat-eating, originally important to men because it connected them to menstrual mental life, is something women were likely to have controlled because of its effects on their own bodies, not solely as part of a collective sex-strike to gain more protein.

I am five years old, and my teenage brother works in the butcher shop of a huge department store in Chicago, where we live. One Saturday night, he brings home a Porterhouse steak, and the ensuing meal is a ceremonial occasion for the whole family, and especially for my hunting-oriented father.

What I remember about the meal is the way the meat was cooked. My mother and sister demanded their portions be small and very well done, without a trace of pink moisture showing. They covered their thin leathery pieces with black pepper. In contrast, and with much proud noise, my father and brother had their thick pieces rare, barely seared, with red blood running over the plate. I was offered no piece of my own, as both sides competed for my favor. And though I ate bites from all contributors, I loudly announced my preference for the rare meat, understanding this to be a moment of public gender identification: I was going to be a boy when I grew up.

What strikes me now about the incident are the subtle expressions of horror the women expressed about eating <u>red</u> meat, blood, and the proud relish of the men toward the same bloody substance. My father felt similarly on the subject of hunting; he schemed and waited decades for the opportunity to go deer hunting. He talked about it, read magazines every month about it, polished his rifles, sanded their stocks, oiled their barrels, collected ammunitions and boots, leather jackets and jackknives. Finally, when he was fifty-six, he had the opportunity to go hunting for two weeks, in the mountains of the Southwest. When he returned empty-handed I

133

thought he would be horribly depressed, but he wasn't. The company of men, the long preparations, the trek itself constituted "the hunt" and had given him something he valued.

Hunters worldwide have kept taboos that are precise imitations of those that developed in the world-forming rites of menstruation. In the eagle hunt of the Hidatsa Indians, the hunters would separate from the rest of the tribe and build a small lodge for special ceremonies, which no woman could enter. They would fast each day until midnight, rise at dawn, speak to no one, and look at no one except for the other secluded hunters. Those who caught nothing wouldn't sleep at all, but spent the night in lamentation and prayer. These rites were performed for four days and four nights, lest "the captive eagle . . . get one of his claws loose and tear his captor's hands." [18]

The similarity between this description of eagle hunting and the experience of menstrual seclusion is striking, and it was typical of other hunting taboos and rites. Fishing as well as hunting was restricted by taboo. Whalers of Nootka Sound fasted for a week, separated from women, and—like the menstruant—were regarded as unclean while being accorded the highest respect. Sexual abstinence for a prescribed length of time was also a common restriction. Often the hunter, like the menstruant, had his own utensils and his own fire, and no one else could touch them. Grooming and bathing prohibitions were similar as well. The Thompson Indian hunters did not comb their hair until their expedition had returned. Across North America, hunters could not scratch their heads or bodies except with a special scratching stick. Hunters often could not eat salt, fat or flesh, or food cooked by a woman of menstrual age. Sometimes they could only drink cold water, or only from a special cup.

The connection between hunting practices and menstruation was often explicit. Many peoples believed that a woman's menstrual or postpartum state could so seriously affect the hunt that her husband could not join it while she was in seclusion. In some societies, women adhered to taboo rules of eating or cooking while the hunters were in the wilderness, in order to protect them and ensure a good kill. *Women's blood, in short, ruled the hunt and gave it its fundamental restrictions and rituals.* Moreover, some peoples credited bows and arrows with the capacity to cause a woman to menstruate. That a hunter's implement might cause a woman to begin to bleed, thus endangering him with contamination, was one reason for keeping weapons away from her, for prohibiting her from stepping over them. Very possibly, the same thinking led the Tiwi and others to consider that sexual intercourse brought about menarche. The penis, arrow, spear, and bow were metaformic "pricks" for blood-letting, male causation of menstruation.[19]

Menstrual rite seems as clearly connected to the practice of hunting as it was to rites of birth, death, and healing. The hunter in his abstinence and fasting, his grooming rites, and his approach to blood, endured seclusions that gave him equal status with the women, equivalent rites, equivalent cooperative work, and his own economic contribution. In this way, the man and the woman danced through life together, coordinated with each other's blood rites.

Herding and Blood Sacrifice

If animals were, as is generally believed, domesticated solely for materialist, practical purposes, as sources of food and hides, then by any logic the most edible and easiest to handle would have been drawn into the fold first. But a blood-toothed and dangerous predator, the wild dog, is believed to have been the first creature brought to the hearth. As we know from the stories of Coyote, Jackal, and Wolf, ancient women connected the wild dog both with menstruation and with the creation of the world. It is thus a measure of the irony, the paradox inherent in menstruation and in our

135

being, that the menstrual mind tamed first the very animal that, as a figure of terror and death, woke us into consciousness.

According to the geographer Carl Sauer, animals like the deer, nonthreatening and near to hand, were never domesticated, while the wilder ones, like the boar whose horns make two lunar crescents, were.[20] The motives for domestication were religious, not economic. In Sauer's example, a hunter from a Southeast Asian fishing village brings a wild piglet, pup, or kid home to his wife or mother. The women nurse these infants from their own breasts, the only way that a creature can actually be adopted into the family of another species. They do not eat them, but consider them relatives, bury them with honor, and treat them as revered ancestors. Joseph Campbell relates how tusks of boars were grown into lunar shapes by men of Malekula in Melanesia, who had learned to substitute boars for human sacrifice. His description of blood dripping between the horns of a ritually slain animal is an explicit depiction of earthly "lunar" menstruation.[21]

This interpretation seems to be confirmed when we look further at early patterns of domestication. The ancestor of domesticated cattle was one of the wildest and most feared, a root stock whose hunting required complex organization and great skill. The earliest kept sheep had to have been desired initially for its horizontal spiral horns, for its wooly coat was a later product of breeding in captivity.[22] The first goat domesticated was also the very wildest of the species, the bezoar, an Asiatic mountain goat living in a remote region of the lower Himalayas, in Afghanistan. The hunters had to travel far, climb sheer cliffs, risk their lives to capture its young. They threw their spears as it stood on the highest peak around, a picture of the moon on earth, displaying its crescents. The hunters took the goat through any peril to themselves—like their brothers pursuing the wooly mammoth and the Great Plains buffalo—as a sign of its fundamental connection to their own beginnings as a people. One Great Plains tribe said of the buffalo that they were "women," that women and the buffalo were the same. I think they meant the same spirit, the same creation-religion, the same meta-form. In the pursuit and sacrifice of horned animals, men were learning and participating in the origination rituals of their societies. They were entering the menstrual mind by engaging with blood power, in their own terms, using parallel rites.

▬ ▬ ▬ ▬ ▬ ▬ ▬ ▬ ▬ ▬ ▬ ▬ ▬ ▬ ▬ ▬ ▬ ▬ ▬

Chapter 9

Sex, Matrimony, and Trickster Wolf

B EFORE cars became a central location for courtship behavior, the tree was a popular spot. The young man took the young woman walking, and they spread a cloth under a large tree and ate bread, cheese, and wine. Or he came to her house, bearing flowers, and pushed her back and forth in her swing, which hung from the limb of a huge backyard tree. Or she, more boldly and after displaying the flesh of her leg or bosom, led him on a flirtatious chase into the wood until he caught her at the base of a large tree, and after having sex, he carved their initials in its bark. One of my old family photos is of such a courtship picnic, with three uncles and aunts and my mother and father, all in their early twenties, in 1920 Illinois.

The prehuman ancestress of millions of years ago, with her mother and sisters nearby, sits in the tallest tree she can climb, keeping still so her blood will not draw the family of jackals. Shooed away by nonmenstruating females, the males of her troop who are quickest to learn "no sex at this time" control their powerful impulse to follow her into the tree. These males have entered the beginning human mind. They know not to arouse the dangerous blood smell or walk around the savannah in the vulnerable state of having blood on their penises. They don't even walk under the tree lest a drop of blood fall on them. For both the men and the woman, the more her rites center on re-creating the world, separating the waters, concentrating on not touching her skin, the more dangerously distracting male sexual influence becomes.

When she comes down from the tree, copulation is again welcomed. This pattern continues indefinitely: when she is in seclusion, she cannot look at males, they cannot come near her; and when she emerges from seclusion, she accepts a sexual union, which, as her *cosmetikos* accrues, becomes more elaborate. It takes place in a specially prepared bed, or hut, or grove of trees. He brings a gift.[1] He connects her garb, her makeup and veiling, to sexuality. She is not just emerging; she is alluring; she is transfixing.

The sexual union directly following menarche or any menstruation is *r'tu*—the word means both menstruation and the ritual heterosexual act that follows the woman's emergence from menstrual seclusion. This sex act has become a central mythic union between the genders, the point at which they unite the comprehensions of their parallel blood-based rites. That this special sexual intercourse initially took place under a tree is perhaps remembered in ancient Greek and other Mediterranean traditions calling upon women of all stations to engage in a single act of sacred prostitution, usually taking place in a grove of trees, and understood as a gift to the Mother Goddess. Traditions of prostitution recall other metaforms of creation as well.

In Rome the office of prostitute was from *Lupa*, "she-wolf," the wolf who nursed Romulus and Remus. Her temple harlots were *lupae*, who initiated young men; and her festival of Lupercalia featured orgiastic rites "to insure the year's fertility."[2] Brothels called *lupernaria* spread throughout Europe with the Roman empire, and all over the world it is the prostitute who welcomes strange men into an area.[3] The prostitute's garb represents a tradition older than that of the bride or weef. Her costume of beads, high heels, earrings, and heavy makeup—to employ a popular stereotype—mark her as an emergent menstruant from the age before cloth, before weaving, when *cosmetikos* was made of paint, strings, and loops, not swathes of cloth or matting.

139

In some current customs the prostitute, or "dancer," has a role prior to the bride's that is perhaps reminiscent of the Lupercalian instruction of Roman times. A night or a few nights before the wedding, the men hold a bachelor party and hire her to appear. Like the bride, she may be accompanied by a cake, though her relations to it are comic. Her job is to sexualize the party, if not to have actual sex with the groom, and she is paid money for her service.

Little Red Cap

Menstruation is associated with sex, as well as with healing, death, and the wolf in a European folktale called "Little Red Cap," more popularly known as "Little Red Riding Hood." Although this story was collected by the Grimms in the nineteenth century, long after the earlier European menstrual customs were layered over or altered to conform with feudalism and early industrialism, its menstrual elements are very evident.

A lovely maid is so appreciative of a red velvet cap her grandmother has lovingly made for her that she never takes it off. She is known as "Little Red Cap." One day the maid is sent by her mother to visit her grandmother, who lives secluded in the forest "half an hour from the village."[4] According to her mother's instruction, Little Red Cap takes with her a bottle of wine and some cake in a basket, for her grandmother is ill. She must not leave the path, her mother warns; but as soon as Little Red Cap enters the forest, she meets a wolf, who persuades her to tell him where the grandmother lives. "Her house is under three oaks. You'll know it by the hazel bushes," says the girl, who is then persuaded by the wolf to leave the path to gather flowers for her beloved grandmother. As everyone surely knows, the wolf then runs ahead, tricks the grandmother into letting him in, eats her, and lies in wait for Little Red Cap in the grandmother's stead. When Little Red Cap finally finds her way to the house, she, too, is devoured. A huntsman arrives, and guessing the worst, he cuts open the wolf's belly,

140

helps the women out, and replaces them with stones, which kill the wolf. Little Red Cap restores her grandmother's health with the cake and wine and vows never to stray off the path again.

In menstrual terms, Little Red Cap reaches menarche and is sent to stay with an old relative in a hut in a secluded place away from the village. She is not just any menarchal initiate, however, but a special one who never takes off her red cap. She is the archetypal menstruant, and her story conveys some developments of human ritual understanding.

Her grandmother being ill, Little Red Cap meets death on the path to her house. By getting "off the path," breaking taboo, she lets the Death Wolf in. The story thus connects menstrual rites to both healing and death. Other details reinforce these associations: the number three counts the "death" of the moon. Since the grandmother's house is near three trees, she must be the moon. The wolf eats her, just as Coyote eats the moon in Native American mythology. The trees that shade the grandmother's house are oak trees. The oak was a sacred tree in many places, and in Europe and the Mediterranean, it was associated with, among other things, child sacrifice. Abraham was said to have pitched his tent under an oak, and it was believed that if you cut an oak, your firstborn son would die.[5] Little Red Cap clearly is in danger. A further clue is added with the mention of hazel bushes. "Hazels" was a synonym for hawthorn, called a hagthorn for its long spikes, associated with the Christian crown of thorns. (And hag, besides being a name for the hedge characteristically made of hazel, is also a name for crone, or in this case, "grandmother.") Prechristian sacrifice is implied by the hagthorn's other name, "Lady's meat"—the brilliant red flowers emit a rotten meat odor so distinct as to attract carrion-loving insects to lay their eggs in the petals.[6] Menstruation and death are identified with the grandmother's house in the forest through the very ancient metaform of the tree and the number three.

Enter the huntsman, a traditional mythic rescuer, one who can be thought of as "orderly man," as distinct from "disorderly man," the wolf. The huntsman frees the sacrificial victims by cutting open

141

the wolf and substituting stones. Besides the menstrual lessons about the causes of disease and death, and the healing power of ritual gifts, the story is clearly a cautionary tale of the dangers of forbidden sex. Uncontrolled male sexuality is called "wolf" in this story (and in contemporary speech), and in a French version of the tale Little Red Cap strips to distract the wolf and escapes by telling him she must go outside to relieve herself.[7] We recall again the Dogon story of the red ant mound, where uncontrolled male sexuality is called the act of the "jackal."

Matrimony

At some point, perhaps less than a million years ago, people came to understand that incestuous mating produced birth defects and extinction. The jackal committed his vile act of incest because he was ignorant of consequences. He did not yet have menstrual knowledge, embodied by the red fiber skirt. He was also alone; in the words of the Dogon, he was not "twinned."[8]

Marriage is a way of twinning, of teaching by pairing. With marriage, exogamy rules. To maintain exogamic unions, elaborate signal systems were needed, not only to indicate who was not appropriate for mating, but also to test whether the prospective mate, a stranger, could participate within the social metaform of the bride's family. After the consciousness of incest, the union at the foot of the tree was not just a single sexual exercise. It was a matrimonial contract that, like menstrual seclusion itself, protected the entire band.

A bridegroom brought gifts, proof of his effective position in a social order, and proof of his toolmaking and hunting skills: venison, furs, and fish, bags of salt, strings of carved shells, lunar-horned cattle, strands of red woodpecker scalps, his family stories and songs—whatever the woman's family valued as "price," he brought.

She brought her *cosmetikos*, her paraphernalia—all the household goods, utensils, wares accumulated in millennia of seclusions.

The word "paraphernalia" literally means the "goods brought by a bride" to her marriage, and in earlier tribal life she went directly from the menstrual hut to the marriage hut. Later she would bring her cedar chest, her elaborate clothing, her linens or cottons, her straw mattings. She would bring her cake, her cooking, her ability to wash, to make everything clean. She would bring as well her healing and death rites, her ability to wail and to mourn. For a multitude of peoples, menarche and matrimony were two parts of one long ritual.

A Tiwi Wedding

As described by Jane Goodale, Tiwi marriages were arranged by the mothers-in-law. A woman made a contract with the man who would be her son-in-law even before a daughter had been born. The girl went to her husband when she was ten or eleven; he was usually about fifteen years older than she. He gradually accustomed her to sexual intercourse, which was then believed to induce her menstruation a year or two later. Her husband was thus completely incorporated into the menstrual mind, given the role of prime cause of the bleeding. Her menarchal rites had two parts, one of seclusion in a woman-only encampment, the second a marriage ceremony. At the second ceremony, she herself became a mother-in-law, her father choosing the man who would husband her own daughters. Although we have mentioned elements of both ceremonies in earlier contexts, it is worth examining the rituals as a whole, for together they comprise some of the deepest and oldest metaforms of humanity.

The menstruant was given the special name *murinaleta;* in one account, the girl's companion asked her five times if she had reached that state before receiving the answer "yes." The companion then began to cry. She tied pandanus-vine armbands of mourning to the menstruant after hitting her with the vines to "kill" her. The menstruant was then taken to a new camp in the bush with female relatives and companions. If her husband saw her there, it was formerly believed, he would die. For five to ten days she stayed, and she was allowed to do no gathering of food, no digging of yams, no cooking, no touching of food or water. The containers were lifted to her lips by others; she could do no scratching, light no fires, look upon no water. At the end of her seclusion, she was painted with a red snake and led by the women to the second camp. There, waiting for her, were her father, her husband, and her husband's brothers. The man her father had chosen for her son-in-law might also wait with them:

> When she first arrives she 'sleeps' for a little while under a blanket. As she lies on the ground her father takes an *arawunigiri*, an elaborately carved ceremonial spear with barbs on two sides, and places it between his daughter's legs. He then presents it to the man whom he has selected to be his daughter's son-in-law. The son-in-law calls the spear "wife" and "hugs it just like a wife," . . . If the son-in-law is not present at this time, the girl's father takes the spear to him sometime after the ensuing rituals. The young girl has by this particular ritual become a mother-in-law.
>
> After the girl's father has presented the spear, he takes . . . a 'palm' tree and sets it upright in the ground. The girl's husband and his brothers line up, with the youngest first in line and her husband last. One by one these men take their *tokwiina* (feather balls) and strike the girls' shoulders. She stands there until it is her husband's turn, when she runs away. . . . The husband pursues his wife, and everyone calls out to her, "Look behind you, him your husband." The girl looks back, and her husband catches her by one shoulder and takes her to the 'palm' tree that her father had set upright, where he makes her sit down. Then he and his brothers take up spears and throw them at the tree, and while doing so they "pretend it is a boy or girl . . ."
>
> The husband and his brothers now dance around the sitting girl, and her father comes and lies down on the opposite side of the tree from his daughter. Her husband then marks the tree with a few strokes of an ax. The marked tree is thereafter known as *aplimeti* (translation unknown). The women place feathered pandanus arm ornaments on her. When her redecoration is complete, her father takes her back to the main camp, followed by all the ritual participants, and he once again hands her over to her husband at his camp-

144

fire. The girl and her husband may not talk to each other upon their return, and that night she must sleep on the opposite side of the fire from him. The next morning the husband paints his young wife, and they may again talk to each other."⁹

The menstruant emerged from seclusion directly into a rite that incorporates men. As the Tiwi ceremony indicates, marriage in the earlier metaforms did not—as it does not in much of modern society today—mark the first sex between the couple. Rather, the marriage ceremony marked the woman's emergence into public life wearing the gifts of menstruation as her garments. The two families and other witnesses then reenacted the ideological relationships that had brought their people to the current moment.

A Modern Wedding

A woman wears the badges of the menarchal office when she marries in contemporary society as well: her special attire, her paint, her hair. Her veil is lace now, her train a gleaming lunar trail of fabric rather than a hide or blanket; her scratching sticks are silver hairpins holding her veil in place. The church of her matrimony may contain the marriage tree as columns of plaster and wood; an arch over the altar imitates the canopy of sky; high on the wall light is captured in a "rose window." The woman walks in a stately manner down a red carpet path on her father's arm and with her people in procession to reach the wooden altar platform. She has special female attendants, as the groom has special male ones. Boys from the groom's side wear ceremonial garb, and one of them holds a red pillow on which is the string of binding memory made of gold. An officiant in white robes may give them red wine and round bread. There are readings from a book of origin stories. The congregation is dressed in finery, none of which is allowed to exceed the bride's. The congregation participate by maintaining appropriate silence, attentive stillness, by following the rituals of standing and sitting. We read and sing aloud in concert. The gifts we have

145

brought are piled in their colorful wrappings in a reception room nearby.

The ceremony is followed by feasting, perhaps dancing. There is music and laughter. There is a cake made of metaforms from older times: finely ground meal, eggs, oil, sweetener. It is white and round, in layers that give it a mountain shape. On top stands a miniature scene of bride and groom under an arch. The cutting of the cake is performed jointly by the wedded couple, who feed it to each other. They twine arms to drink from a single cup. After a time of celebration, the couple goes to a special car, humorously decorated (hung with shoes). As they depart, rice is showered on them to bring fertility and prosperity. They drive to a special wedding bed, which may be a rose and red painted room; the cover of the bed is often very decorative. (In older times, it would have been a quilt made by the bride and her female relatives that included cosmological imagery. In older times still, this imagery would have pertained to her place in the cosmos and village and carried astronomical and other data particular to her life.) The groom may carry the bride through the doorway to the bed, or this "not touching the ground" ceremony may be saved for their first entry into the home they will share.[10] The wedding bed itself is raised off the ground and has four posts, perhaps a canopy. In this "grove" the couple consummate their marriage under trees and enter the state known as "honeymoon," the sweetest moon, the new moon of sexual love.

At the one wedding I have attended, when the flower girls appeared at the back of the church, and when the bride, gleaming white on her parent's arm, began her walk down the red carpet path, I did what I'm told women always do, I wept. (So did my girlfriend's father.) We see her, the moon walking on earth, and she is our eternity and our mortality, and we both adore and mourn. We see the groom's unease, and his human courage to combine with the terrible mystery of life and death, his desire to conform to the restrictions of fidelity and paternity. We see his fragility, and hers, and their nobility; they stretch us backward and forward in time. We call the reason for our weeping "her beauty."

Remnants of ancient menarchal rites run through our formal wedding practices, for they are originally the same rite. The groom may not see the bride or her gown before the moment of her emergence at the wedding; she is kept hidden from him. She then arrives out of her seclusion, splendidly washed, combed, and dressed. When her new husband toasts her, he may break the wine glass after drinking—as utensils were broken in earlier blood rites. He has been invited into the menarchal pattern. He lifts the veil to kiss her, or he paints her face; he brings significant gifts. If he carries her across the threshold, it is because in ancient times she was forbidden to touch the ground. Hereafter, when they dress up to go out dancing, she will wear high heels that lift her off the ground, and he will feel both tender toward this vulnerability, and uneasy at the sharpness of the spikes.

Marriage displays the whole cosmogony of menstruation in one rite. The participants—who are not related to each other—demonstrate their comprehension of the essential metaform, which will hold together regardless of the fate of this particular marriage. This is because a marriage represents more than a promise between two individuals. Rather, it ties together the two genders, as well as the two families, in shared understanding of one cosmogony whose roots are menstrual, whose consummation is sexual, and whose purpose is cultural.

Bridal Dress

The bride's dress in Europe was formerly red. In places with a rich village life, such as Turkey, the bridal dress is still fundamentally red, with other colors and rich embroidery layered on top. Before the Ottoman Empire outlawed the fez, this high felt red cap was a prominent part of women's garb, used to lift the veil high and hold it in place. The veils were not filmy but solid and deeply colored

147

cloth, often red, and fell below the waist, a wall behind which neither the bride's face nor the shape of her body could be seen.[11]

A common headdress shape was the cone. Many menstrual seclusion huts also took the form of a cone. The Middle Eastern bride
and the bride of feudal Europe, hung with fabrics from head to
foot, her headpiece towering above her, can be said to carry with
her the menstrual hut. We can find startlingly similar patterns in
the ritual garb of a variety of cultures. In the Yukon valley, a
menstruant wore a long robe with a large hood, and among the
Thompson Indians, her face was painted red, a heavy blanket
swathed her entire body, and a conical hat of fir branches reached
her breast. African mediums impersonate the goddess Oyá, draping
themselves from head to foot in layer after layer of richly decorated
cloth until they resemble walking houses.[12] Bao Lord describes yet
another elaboration in *Spring Moon: A Novel of China*.[13] Dressed
entirely in red, with a jeweled headdress, the bride was placed in a
red sedan chair that was completely sealed. She was carried to her
wedding and set down outside the ceremonial hall, where the men
gathered and sang three songs to her, songs that were tests of her
character. Then they tapped three times on the chamber and she
emerged, while everyone cried, "The bride, the bride," over and
over. She walked on a red carpet to the wedding ceremony, where
the groom lifted her red silk veil. The veil, the hut, and the sedan
chair are all variations of the same form. They are containers of
her power.

We have seen that marriage rites, whether ancient or modern,
are an extension of menarchal rites. The ancestress bled, was secluded, went through the transformations of *cosmetikos,* and
emerged for a feast and procession that ended in or included sexual
union. In the enactment of the incest taboo, the groom needed to
be formally incorporated into her family, and into the menarchal
metaform. The red fiber skirt of the first Word became in some
areas a full length red dress. The bride might wear not only her
menarchal cap, but also a veil over her face, head, or entire body;
through the veil only one male, the bridegroom, might go. With

148

such rites, powerful sexual instincts were brought under human control, so that we have come to use sexuality in uniquely human ways, and for far more than reproduction. Tantrism, the sexual arts of health, pleasure, psychism, and spiritual intimacy, are taught in India, many parts of Asia, and in the United States, and include lesbianism as a healthy human activity. I remember lesbian lovers with whom I have shared moments of spontaneous and exultant love and trust as we painted stripes on our bare torsoes with our own fresh menstrual blood. We were "blood sisters," initiating each other into women's power, without words or any outside eye gauging the meaning of our rite.

Cosmetikos

The body arts that taught us how to think and act as human beings underlie our everyday lives. We are so dependent on them we hardly give them a thought. *Cosmetikos* gave us the body paint, ornamentation, and clothing that so strikingly differentiate us from other creatures. It also provided the paraphernalia that became kitchenware and household goods. More surprisingly, *cosmetikos* created our manners and formalities at table; our various methods of cooking, brewing, and preserving; and even the nature of the foodstuffs we gather and grow. Most important, *cosmetikos* gave us the ideas with which we regulate our bodies, chiefly in terms of paired opposites that are also polarities of the menstrual cycle (bleeding/not bleeding) and the lunar cycle (dark moon/light moon). Some of the pairings of *cosmetikos* include unclean/clean, sick/well, inauspicious/auspicious, hot/cold, raw/cooked, unlucky/lucky, and cursed/blessed. The word "cursed" is still directly related to menstruation, in common jargon; and the word "blessed" is as well, deriving as it does from German "blood-song," blessing. Both sides of the equation derive from menstruation, not just the "negative" or dark moon, but the full moon as well. Menstruation has created so much of what we are, including our capacity to judge abstract qualities of good and bad.

149

The institutions of *cosmetikos* are worldwide. Even if human culture shrank to three people who spoke three different languages, they would probably recall how to handle fire, make a knife, a pot of gathered foods, clothing, body decoration, huts, a chair. They would understand these forms whether or not they discussed their meanings. But to remember mathematics, to tell stories, to solve geometry problems—for these things, *cosmetikos* might not help them. They would need to bring the set of arts and sciences I call narrative, which began in *cosmetikos* but developed into a unique set of metaforms. Are the narrative metaforms connected to my rejected cosmetic case? Only if you add my mother's sewing kit, and a knife or sharp flint.

Part Three

. . . A N D . . .
Narrative Metaform

Chapter 10

■■■■■■■■■■■■■■■■■■■■■■■■■■■

Number, Orientation, and the Shapes of Light

I am eight and in the third grade. At night I lie awake, feeling
bad. I even imagine sneaking silently into the kitchen so I can
stab myself with the butcher knife. The reason? because I cannot understand arithmetic. Yet I'm supposed to be smart—smart
is the one thing I have going for myself.

My father uses numbers to work in the steel factory, to measure
the dimensions of its products. In the little dresser drawer near his
bed, three sets of calipers lie in their soft bed of blue velveteen
inside a stiff black pouch, which folds close around them like the
covers of a black and holy book. My craftsman father is very proud
and careful of his calipers. I am not to play with them, and though
I break this admonition in all other instances, I respect my father's
calipers, only using them under his instruction, to draw circles.

My father's narrations incorporate number in detail. A pistol is
never just a pistol. A gun is not just a rifle. No—it is named in
detail, with numbers: a 45-caliber semiautomatic Smith and Wes-
son with a seven-shot magazine, a quarter-inch bore, a double barrel, a nine millimeter shell, a ten-inch barrel, a split-second action,
a $639 price tag, a 1940 year of manufacture, a World War I his-
tory, and "a kick that will take both yer arms off."

I notice as I grow older that if I don't have numbers and names
right, the men will stop talking, snort at me, and then continue
without me. Precision of number as well as name is how they keep

track of who is paying attention, who is "smart" enough to stay in the conversation game with them. Number tells us how much to believe a story.

My mother, who hates guns, withdraws from the dialogue and then the room while these conversations go on. In her little kitchen there is almost no measurement. Nearly everything she cooks comes from a can or is prepackaged and presliced. Her sewing basket, equipped with two spools of thread, a package of needles and a thimble, is used only for darning socks: "That's all I know of sewing." Often no one believes my mother's stories, she stumbles over details and dates, can't recall addresses, loses track of weeks, and months. Without number, she can't find her place in stories.

In earlier times, when my mother retreated to the kitchen, she would have joined in an ongoing discussion between women regarding the size of pickle barrels, weight of the herring fillets, age of the children, teaspoons of vinegar. Cups of flour would have mixed with the number of stitches in the quilt, number of colors in the rug, yardage of the bolts of cloth, timing of the plantings, number of seeds, and dispositions of the harvest and the number of days until the baby's birthday. Her meagre sewing basket would have held more than socks. She would have participated in the rich traditions of women's sewing, knitting, crocheting, quiltmaking, netmaking, macrame, weaving, plaiting, basketry, and pottery—with their geometry, mathematics, color sense, and storytelling, splendid ceremonial occasions. Still further back in the women's tradition were astronomical divination, card and palm reading, the Tarot, the architecture of houses and farm buildings, and before that, the temples. Any part of this once would have been my mother's inheritance, but in her life, none of it was. In her understanding, men had created the world, and its numbers. She had inherited the industrial revolution, which scooped up all of her arts and treasures and carried them into factories outside the home and outside of her charge.

154

The Menstruantas Calendar

What is the story of number? According to Alexander Marshack, who decoded the earliest known human markings on bones and stones as notations of lunar months, people approached number with a sense of groupings, rather than with any linear sense of sequence.[1] As I imagine it, the original number must have been what we now call a month, a unit synchronized to menstruation. Within this unit, other units began to take shape: a set of three units meaning "dark moon," a set of fifteen units meaning "half moon," and so on. From long before the earliest known numerical notation, people must have been thinking in terms of groups of numbers, using number as story—plot, character, and relationship.

At first, the menstruant, whenever she secluded during the dark of the moon and emerged at the new moon, *was* the calendar. She marked a definitive, externally visible, unit of time, the month (*moon*th) as synchronized within the human body:

> Chinese women established a lunar calendar 3000 years ago, dividing the celestial sphere into 28 stellar "mansions" through which the moon passed. Among the Maya of central America, every woman knew "the great Maya calendar had first been based on her menstrual cycles." Romans called the calculation of time mensuration, i.e., knowledge of the menses; menstrua is a grammatical form of menstruus, monthly; mensura is measurement. Gaelic words for "menstruation" and "calendar" are the same: *miosach* and *miosachan*. The new-moon sabbaths of ancient Latium were *kalends,* possibly related to the Aryan name of Kali.[2]

The Hindu goddess was the goddess of the dark of the moon. She was connected to blood of all kinds and was often portrayed with dreadful face painted red, an uncontrollable deadly force, though her religion is extremely complex and she is also Mother Kali, Kali Ma, Sara Kali. However, she is crone and dark moon more than most goddesses, and she is a trinity, so the number three—the number of the dark moon—belongs to her.

155

. . . A N D . . .

The ancestress cloistered herself in her hut, gathering the paraphernalia of her *r'tu* around her: her blood-drawing flint, her
scratching stick, her little white, red, or black marking stones, her
bird bone straw. Sooner or later she would scratch the units of her
correspondence with the moon into written form. Such calendric
markings have been found in the south of France, on two hollow
eagle bones dating from the Upper Paleolithic period of 12 to
15,000 B.C.E. One of these bones investigated by Marshack, long,
hollow, and three-sided, was also grooved to be a whistle.[3] Without
the groove, it could have been a straw, as perhaps the second bone
was. Remembering that hollow eagle-bone straws were used in
menstrual rite to "separate the waters," it makes sense that a lunar
calendar was kept on eagle bones. The eagle surely was at times
imagined as the moon itself, as other large birds have been, or as a
cloud and therefore a bringer of rain, the menstruation of the sky.
The eagle shows a striking white moon shape on its tail in flight,
and is a predator associated with blood. It is also the supreme spirit
bird for many peoples of the North American continent.

One of the eagle wing bones examined by Marshack contained
a six-month lunar calendar on two of its sides. Through careful
microscopic examination of the strokes, Marshack deduced patterns marking the lunar phases: quarter, half, crescent, dark, crescent again. The marks on one bone were in distinct groups of 7 and
15, then 29, then 25 plus 4, suggesting direct observation of the
moon's changes. Calendar markings from a similar age have been
found on stone disks, breast- and vulva-shaped stones, and other
objects signifying the feminine.[4]

The question of which gender made which specific Paleolithic
markings or drawings is largely unanswerable and probably irrelevant, since both genders have had to practice these arts in order to
learn time's dimensions. Through parallel menstrual rites of the
hunt and of animal and human sacrifice, men were coordinated to
the lunar cycle. They went out hunting the eagle and brought its
bones back to the village. They, too, sat in seclusion in lonely places
with bones and stones, a flint knife, pondering the shape-shifting

156

light above their heads. But the menstruant, having the most direct connection with the lunar cycle, would surely have been the first to know; she had motive, method, and opportunity to be the originator of lunar notation.

Sacred Number Enacted and Embodied

Menstrual seclusion rites enact and make sacred specific numbers, and it is this specificity of attention to *groups* of numbers connected to lunar events that makes the science of numbers so much larger than simple sequential counting could ever have been. The group of numbers used in a tribe's particular seclusion rites varied, even among tribes living in the same areas. But whether the number of days of menarche was 3, 4, 5, 6, 7, 8, or 100, whether it stood for one month or seven years, its significance was defined by the central physical rite. Not only was the menstruant secluded, she was secluded for a particular number of days and nights. And whatever number was specified for menarche, the same number was sacred in other tribal rites and was recognized by the tribe as their "sacred number."[5] Thus people studied number as if it were name, a group of letters adding up to a sacred, creative word: Three, Five, Seven.

I'm suggesting—keeping in mind Marshack's expression "time-factored thought"—that our ancestors may have learned to think numerically through their recognition of relationships between groups of numbers that were also units of time measured through menstrual rite. Perhaps this explains the fact that although many tribes described in the nineteenth-century accounts did not seem to have words for very high numbers—no idea of "thousand," for instance—they nevertheless had complex numerology in their social customs, dances, and crafts, paying strict attention to ritual numbers and "proper" timing. It seems likely that ancestral people began by using number ceremonially, as ratio, as relationship—not as quantity, not even as sequence.

Menstrual rite measured durations of time that were witnessed

157

by the people as a whole, beginning of course with the menstruant's relation to the presence and absence of light. Logically, the original sacred number would have been one menstrual cycle, which was commonly counted as twenty-eight days—twenty-five of the moon's light and three of the moon's dark—or thirty days.

It is not important that the actual number of days in the menstrual cycle may have been slightly more or that the moon is by modern calculations completely dark for only one day, not three. Early humans, just beginning to express their consciousness of time, were not so much observing the sky in the interest of precise counting as they were closely connecting its patterns to their bodies, spirits, and stories. Three days for the moon's menstruation is a closer entrainment to women's bleeding than is one day. Three is worldwide the number associated with death, with completion, and with birth, all of which are also equated with the moon's disappearance and reappearance. Three days for the dark of the moon remained the convention over much of the world as late as the founding of the Jewish calendar, which retains it.

Even today, long after the practice of a three-day seclusion, number lingers in menstrual lore: "Whenever they had their very first period, my mom sat with each of her daughters for about ten minutes on the third stair, so that they would always have regular periods. She was born in 1939, and this was in Bulacan Province, in the Philippines."[6]

Number as Ornament

Although I have no explicit evidence, I believe the earliest notation of number must have been on the human face; where men, especially, could see it. Perhaps, like Snake, numerical *cosmetikos* represents "Female Instructing Principle." The connection of three to menstrual *cosmetikos* was most dramatic and artful in the practice of chin tattooing, the widespread use of three vertical lines to mark the passage of a woman through menarche into adulthood. As we

158

have seen, the highly visible, emblematic chin tattoo served to protect the vulnerable mouth.

But the lip bar with three evenly spaced "dribble" lines running from it may also have imprinted the sacred number three on the whole tribe—the unit of time of the moon's disappearance as related to the female vulva. Turned up on its right side this mark is a squared-off version of how we write the number three today.

Cosmetikos, as I have said, begins with an embedding of the significant mark or shape in the flesh itself, then later the same mark is painted on the skin, and later still, painted or indented on another surface—cloth, bread, or a pot—that is metaformic of human flesh. Over the course of time and cultural additions, *cosmetikos* migrated out from the flesh onto other surfaces. Thus, while in 1936, an Aleutian woman would have cut the tri-bar line into her daughter's chin with flint or a thorn, a Moroccan bride would have her chin marked with three lines of charcoal, and in Central Asia, a smith might have worked the number three into a design of silver and gems to be worn as a delicate veil over the married woman's mouth whenever she went outside.

The work of Marija Gimbutas, an archaeologist specializing in woman-centered cultures of prehistoric Europe, seems to confirm the significance of the number three.[7] One of the female figures she describes, from Mycenae 1300 B.C.E., has a serpent head. Its mouth consists of a bar with three lines coming down the chin. Patterns of three lines are also found on woman-shaped pots and figurines from the Upper Paleolithic. Since the pots are goddess figures—in my view, representations of the collective menstruant—at one time these marks may have been chin tattoos incised on the faces of real women on the European continent. Gimbutas considers these tri-lines and similar numerical lines on clay and stone to have been the early basis of writing. If so, the notation of significant numbers—particularly in the Northern Hemisphere, the number three—could have begun as incisions on the face representing the achievement of menstrual status.

159

Gimbutas also points out the significance of the large number of V's or chevrons identified as vulva marks. The V was painted and incised on early goddess figures as the vulva, possibly also as an early method of drawing the crescent moon or representing one lunar day. Some of the pot marks seem to be an entire statement of time. In one instance the chevrons can be seen as the waning and waxing moon, with the space between being menstruation, the dark, chaos, nothing: ⟨ ⟩. In another example, the waning and waxing crescents surround three vertical lines: ⟨|||⟩. Perhaps the three-line chin tattoos are merely a remnant of a great complexity of numerical incisions worn by people in the distant past.[8]

The menstruant kept time with her seclusions, and women kept number on their bodies. They taught us what time it is, and how to think proportionately; they taught us how to connect events together, to add them up. They taught us the power of the essential metaphor implicit in the connective word "and." They also taught us where in the world we are.

The Menstruant as Compass: Orientation

The word "orientation" comes from Latin and means "east." It is related to both *oriri*, "to rise," and *rivus*, "stream." The word "cardinal," meaning primary, and applied both to the four directions and to elemental numbers, also means a woman's hooded cloak, formerly made of scarlet material. In the derivations of these words, I am reminded that in many menarchal rites, the menstruant emerged from her seclusion at dawn. This act faced her toward the east. It must have been part of *r'tu* from the earliest division of light from dark—mythologically speaking, the second "world" or level of consciousness after the ancestress noticed that predators were attracted to her blood. Since in so many seclusion rites her emergence, as an act of world formation, was at dawn, she can be said to have "created" east.

Later the seclusion hut itself would have been built so that its opening faced east for her emergence. She had become a ritual

160

compass. The hut and her emergence from it established the original cardinal direction and the basis for orientation. Her reappearance from the hut with the reappearance of light was public, with her family and perhaps her entire village present for the feast. This meant that everyone would observe her orientation, her "eastness." That orientation would have passed over into other rites as they developed, and people would have learned direction by imitating the menstrual emergence toward the east at dawn. The keeping and display of direction became one of the central organizing principles for all human ritual and was integrated into tribal and village life to a degree modern minds can scarcely imagine.[9] Thus, in some menarchal rites, the menstruant was required to dance all night long, facing east, often shaking a rattle.[10] Women companions stood on each side to hold her when she was tired, for she must not stop. Other menarches included a race, in imitation of the sun or moon. The emergent menstruant led the race—she *was* the light—running in its course from east to west, and then returning. She could not look back. In Kinaaldá, the elaborate menarchal ceremony of the Navajo, she runs at dawn and at noon toward the east in a clockwise direction, around a tree or other significant plant, and then runs back to the hogan. Her companions give chase, careful to let her win. She embodies east and west and the path, or course (*rita*), that light follows. West was reinforced in many mourning rites. For example, the relatives or the healer would leave a sick person's hut by the "back door," that is, toward the west, the direction of death for many peoples. Special holes were torn in the west walls to remove a corpse from a house. Since east represented renewal, birth, revelation, and source of light, in many origin stories west became the place of death, disappearance of light, and onset of dark.

The Sacred Shapes of Light

The circle, arc, straight line, triangle, cone, square, and rectangle are used in the mathematical method of reasoning called "geome-

161

try" (from *geo,* "earth," and *metron,* "measure") because eventually combination of these shapes with number led to the ability to measure the surface of the earth, the circumference of the equator, the distance from equator to pole, the distance between the earth and the moon and sun, and the circumference of both. The shapes used for these calculations were worn on the menstruant's body as *cosmetikos.* They ordered the cosmos by imitating its sky shapes and protected the sacred vulva by honoring its pubic triangle. For millennia, such forms as parallel lines, the circle, triangle, and crescent had been carved, painted, and inserted into the skin, arched into eyebrows, woven in string designs, baskets, and garments, constructed in sacred huts and lodges, and drawn on the walls of caves and cowsheds in coordination with menstrual *r'tu.* Somewhere back in the millions of years that the ancestress sat shedding her apehood in her seclusions, her mother cut her lip and inserted a piece of *round* shell to protect her from harm. In expressing the correspondence between menstruation and significant shapes, the menstrual mind gathered the fundamentals of what would become geometry. When sacred shape and sacred number migrated away from *cosmetikos* and were applied to movement, architecture, landscape, and story, we had the beginnings of the sciences of surveying, engineering, navigating, and "pure" geometry. But as with number, the primary shapes of geometry were metaformic. They were held sacred and learned through *r'tu.*

Almost everywhere, people perform rites after first forming themselves into a circle. This is not a "natural" pattern; few animals make circular formations. Here on earth there was nothing to draw people to the circular shape. The circle was in the sky, the light that came and went, the light whose habits and whose shapes the menstruant imitated. Early peoples devised ingenious methods of studying the circle: rouge spots were painted on cheeks; dots, circles, and round shapes were engraved on the body; round lip pegs and disks were fitted. The people ate from round plates and bowls, used round mats, round baskets. Plazas and other places of public ceremony were laid out in a circle, as were many villages.

Plains Indian women arranged the tribe's tipis in a circle of wholeness. Dwellings themselves articulated the circle—round houses, huts, tents. Hoop games, games played in a ring, circle dances, and the making of round drums—whose shape imitates the moon and whose beats make use of rhythmic timings—all reinforced the image. And everywhere on earth people now make the circle—in games and dances, around campfires, in churches, and in hundreds of other ways.

The moon, as we've seen, is the source of a number of sacred shapes. Fullness, the circle, became the philosophical idea of wholeness because the moon goes through its cycle of less whole, vanished, and then increasingly whole to the point of completion again. Crescent forms dominated the adornment of tribal people all over the world, especially horns, tusks, nails, and claws. These shapes were worn all over the body. Tusks and even slender horns were used as nose ornaments. Horns were a prominent feature of the costumes of holy people, shamans, and of mediums impersonating deities—from the West African goddess Oyá, whose horns are those of the buffalo, to the singles and double-horned gods of the Pueblo peoples and the buffalo spirits of the Plains tribes. In the West, the crescent is singled out on the female body when polish is applied to every part of the fingernail except the little lighter colored area near the cuticle, an area known as the "moon." And croissants, French crescent rolls, are still sometimes called "the moon's teeth." [11]

The gathering of metaforms that imitated the shapes of the moon's changes led people to subdivide the unit "month" into halves, thirds, and the measure we use so often in the West, "quarters." The specific designations might vary, for they did not need to be based in an exact number of days, but rather on the appearance of the crescent, the half, and the full moon. Nevertheless, recognition of a semicircle as the shape of a moon halfway through its cycle represents the idea of the fraction: half, the even division of parts. Quarter is a further extension of this important geometric (originally lunametric) perception.

163

Dividing the lunar cycle into quarters enabled people to quarter the entire visible sky as well. The fact that both moon and sun follow a similar east-west course, so that the path of light appears to "cut" the sky in half, would have expressed further the idea of proportional division. For some peoples, the fundamental directions east-west were sufficient, but most others quartered the sky and established four directions. The Tibetans coordinated the moon's phases with the directions: east was crescent, west was full moon; south, the half moon, and north, the dark of the moon.

Once this scheme of measurement was in place, it could be transferred to the earth. Mythology from many places insists that measurement began in the sky and then fell or otherwise came to live on earth. Imperial China used the sacred number nine—the sum of the four directions in the sky, the four directions on earth, and the emperor in the center, representing all human society. Many other peoples took three as the sky's number and four as the earth's, in a sacred number that combined them: seven.

The idea of dividing the sky or the moon into parts was practiced by the ritual cutting of the lunar pie or cake by the emergent menstruant or by a parallel menstruant, such as a priest. Round cakes in many religious services are carefully cut by quartering or are decorated in cross marks, especially on those occasions associated with sun/moon coordinations.

Number and My Own Mind

In the sixth grade, the veil that has hidden numbers from me suddenly lifts with geometry. The relationship of number to shape, of ratio to proportion, of proportion to balance and esthetic—this I understand well and get great pleasure from. I don't excel at solving problems, but I comprehend the principles. Then with algebra, the curtain falls again. The relationship of number to itself baffles me completely.

I know only one girl who "gets" higher mathematics—my best friend, Francine, whose Arab ancestors discovered and developed algebra and whose mother as well as father is a technician in rocket engineering at White Sands Proving Grounds. Mathematics is not an abstraction to her, and trigonometry is a delight. Her parents give her the patterns of mathematics as my own give me the patterns of poetry.

I want measurement through number, orientation, and shape to be my own. Simple addition and subtraction become my mother's when at forty-two she goes to work outside the home, as a photographer's assistant. She uses her salary to pay the gas, water, and light bills, and sometimes for food and rent too. She gets great and obvious satisfaction from paying these bills, partly because of the security of having household money in her own control, for my father is periodically likely to drink up and gamble away his own salary.

I also believe she gets satisfaction simply from using number in her daily life, from writing down amounts, adding and subtracting the slender figures on paper, and then again in her head when doling out money for me to go to the store. "Three peaches, the smallest container of baking soda, and a quart of milk," she says, her eyes rolling to the ceiling as she mentally calculates the probable cost before fishing a bill and change and wrapping my small fist around them. "Don't forget to add it up when the checker does," she says. "Sometimes they make a mistake." I consider the chore a success if I am accurate within five cents of the checker's conclusion.

In the absence of a strong feminine tradition, and without much access to the male tradition, my mother's mind drifts away from us, at times completely. I am afraid this will happen to me as well. But, like her, having lost number in the sudden abstraction of algebra, I find it again when I go to work. Almost all my first jobs require using a cash register, making change, and immediately addition and subtraction are back in my life. Long before turning me out into the world at seventeen, my mother carefully teaches me how to manage a bank account, to fill out the checks and keep track of the amounts.

I am proud of this skill that my mother did not have until half way through her long life, and that my grandmother did not have at all. My mother stresses that the difference between having money of one's own—however small the amount—and having none was the difference between survival and hell.

When at twenty-one I spend a year training as a medical laboratory technician, I am thrilled with the amount of measurement and math required. Chemical substances are not only named but given numeric value, valence, based in their molecular structure. Once again, what has been a veil of secrecy lifts as I take the calibrated tubes (glass straws!) and vessels in my hands, and mix exact amounts of human blood and chemical toward a particular end—the proportion in millimeters of white cells to red indicating the difference between leukemia and not leukemia for the very real man sitting in the examining room. Stopwatch in hand, pipette in mouth, sharp smell of sulphuric acid in nose, charts and graphs fixing my eye, I revel in the measurements of my occupation despite my dislike for the more mechanistic, fragmented, and unjust aspects of Western medicine. At least, I feel, I have a piece of numerical mind.

Cat's Cradle, Parallel Lines, and Triangles

The geometric forms based, not in circles, but in straight and parallel lines—the cross, the square, and the triangle—cannot be based in the moon's shapes or motions. Yet mythology and art history tell us that straight-line forms such as triangles are very much related to menstruation and women's arts. Where did they come from?

We don't have to go far to find a method by which women in the most distant past could have been drawing complex parallel line figures without using any materials other than a bit of vine and their two hands. Cat's cradle is a game played by looping a continuous cord over the fingers of both hands held apart with palms facing, making patterns in the cord by changing the relationship

166

of the loops. Girls in my culture still play cat's cradle. (I didn't, of course—that was "girl stuff.") People worldwide play string games—in the South Pacific, whole families do—and in nineteenth-century Africa, it was a test of intelligence.[12]

Women of the Yirrkalla people of Australia tell how the two creation sisters, the Wawilak Sisters, originated cat's cradle and the use of string. As the two sisters looked at each other's menstrual blood, each made a loop of the other's blood and put it around her neck. They had become blood sisters in the most fundamental sense of that expression.[13] In the myth, the Snake of synchroneity appeared when the younger sister saw the blood of birth on the elder's vulva and started her own period—and she was making a cat's cradle design at the same time. A Yirrkalla cat's cradle figure is titled "Menstrual blood of three women." The loops are made around the thumb, forefinger, and little finger of each hand, forming three interconnected "streams." The figure as a whole contains triangles and a central diamond shape, and of course, it calls attention to synchrony between menstruation and the number three. (It is not surprising, then, that the triangle figure is associated with the vulva.) In Yirrkalla society only the women do cat's cradle. The men must walk past a woman looping the string with their eyes averted. Women of the aboriginal tribes are said to "own the string."[14]

In the mythology of geometry, two sisters comprehended the synchrony of their blood flows as "Snake" and also saw that the strings of blood and the navel string and strings of vine *were all the same.* They expressed the correspondence by creating figures from a hand-held net of string—the cat's cradle—understood metaform-ically as "strings of blood." When the string formations of cat's cradle are imitated in chalk or carving, they are *drawings,* ways of attracting and capturing spirits toward specific purposes. (Art critics in modern times describe art's spirit-catching attributes in terms of proportion, balance, form, and energy.)

The string held taut in the hands taught us to use forms based in straight lines, parallel and intersecting: triangles, trapezoids, rectangles. These forms were transferred from string to other human "drawings." In all the crafts and ornaments of humankind, geometric designs served as protection against the disintegrative power of menstrual consciousness of disaster. Women painted and tatooed the figures on their own and also on the men's bodies, as they do still today along the Amazon River and other places. Their scratching sticks and combs were decorated with significant lines and triangles. Once they learned to weave cloth, they dyed the geometric figures in it, giving the cloth of Africa and South America, as prime examples, its exquisite artfulness. The geometric pottery painting and beadwork of American Indians gave their societies their distinctive esthetic. In Scandinavian and other folk cultures, linear formality of design was the rule. In old African cultures, triangular and circular forms, usually painted by the women, dominated the external ornamentation and design of villages and buildings.

The sun, or light, is also related to the cat's cradle game, which for its original users was far more than a recreation. The string figure was a method of affecting the external world. The Eskimo of Iglulik used cat's cradle figures to slow the sun's disappearance during the fall months, "to catch him in the meshes of the string," while farmers used string figures to influence their crops.[15]

Combinations of Sacred Number and Sacred Shape: Pi

When sacred number and sacred form were combined, the science of formal measurement resulted, and the relationships, sizes, and distances between the bodies in the sky and the earth began to be determined. The sacred rope (the umbilical Snake), with a peg or rod to center it, could be used to draw a perfect circle on the ground, of which the rope was the radius. The circle could be halved by any two opposed points on its circumference, and the line of splitting was Tiamat, *diameter*. When the sacred number three was applied to the circular form and to its rope diameter, a "magic" formula emerged that operated for any circle of any size:

168

three multiplied times the diameter equals the circumference. Stated mythically, application of the dark of the moon (three) to the half moon (diameter) produces the full moon (circumference). This formula could have used units that consisted of ropes of equal lengths; it did not require number units. In folk medicine, an act must often be repeated three times, and that symbolic equation might be stated thus: perform a metaformic action (diameter) three times (dark moon) to achieve healing (wholeness, full moon).

A second formula can be pulled from a similar combination of elements: the sum of the radius multiplied times itself times the sacred number three equals the area within the circle. The elements of the formulas—the full moon shape, divided into light/dark or aboveworld/belowworld by the rope diameter, which is multiplied by the dark moon three—lead again to the fullness of the circle with its circumference and area. The application of sacred number to sacred form enabled early thinkers to capture the measure of light and dark in a new rope web, just as they had been "capturing light" for millennia in cat's cradle figures and witches knots.

Formulas based in three applied to the circle were used by temple, ziggurat, and pyramid builders in China, Mesopotamia, and Egypt.[16] More recently, the sacred number three became refined to a decimal value, by convention now, 3.14 or 3 1/7. Greeks called this number *pi;* they learned its formula thousands of years after the earlier architects of Stonehenge, Babylon, and Egypt had incorporated it into their temples and pyramids. In China, the *Pi*-dragon retained the formula's association with the (vaginal) serpent. I find I remember it better if I also think of my mother's cherry pie.

The most prominent numbers *of cosmetikos*—measuring the separations of menstrual creation (five), the days of lunar death (three), and the directions of the oriented earth (four)—when applied as a ratio, a relationship, make a triangle with a very special quality: one of its angles is 90 degrees. With this formula, walls and floors can be perfectly squared; the relationship of the horizontal to the vertical can be perfectly squared. Babylonian architects used a knotted rope divided into 3-4-5 proportions to align their buildings. And in Egypt, not only did the royal builders and master architects use it, but even ordinary Egyptian farmers used 3-4-5 knots to mark out their fields and reestablish boundaries after the annual Nile flood.

The Greek mathematician Pythagoras, who studied in Egypt, separated the proportionate structure of the old 3-4-5 triangle from its knotted umbilical rope and from its practical uses, teaching its proportions as a purely mental and spiritual exercise to his students. Pythagoreans and Platonists believed the triangle to be the fundamental building block of the cosmos. Since Pythagoras was the first to bring the form to Western consciousness, he was long believed to have "created" it.

How long ago our ancestors first set a pole upright from the ground and used the angle it made to measure the sun's shadow, and from this, to begin to calculate the dimensions of the earth, moon, and sun, and their relative distances from each other, is probably unknowable. But clearly, peoples long before the Greek mathematicians possessed the fundamental elements of this kind of measurement. Mythology credits both genders, as it should. Egyptian hieroglyphs portray the goddesses Isis and Nepthys as measurers; they often hold a rope between them.[17] A graphic description of the right triangle is particularly apt: the two short sides are formed by the body of a long thin serpent; the hypothenuse is the leaning body of an Egyptian King, his erect penis centered. The glyph thus credits the sacred 3-4-5 triangle to the female tradition of Snake, coupled with the royal male. In the Book of the Dead, a hooded serpent is consistently part of the glyph for the many goddesses named in the text.

Sacred numbers remained attached to the deities as they developed in the Greek pantheon, and also the pantheon of the Macumba religion in West Africa. Hera's number was nine; to goddesses connected to the underworld and death—Hecate and Kali, for example—belonged the sacred number three. Number *is* narrative, for number establishes relationship in space and time. Number thus gave us a capacity to tell sequential stories—stories with a specific past or future, with relationships between significant characters, or "names," units of sacred meaning. Our capacity to repeat in fixed numbers enabled us to find significance in other fixed repetitions, as when the cock crows three times. The meta-forms of number, orientation, and shape have given us certain key elements of our stories: when, where, who, how many, how long? The lunar-menstrual ratios of number and shape gave us ideas of partialness and wholeness. In short, the connective capacity of metaform gave us story itself, the connective word "and." The moon is secluded *and* so is the menstruant.

Chapter 11

The Making of the Goddess

Royal Red Regalia

The problem with everything that accrued to the power of blood is that it all had to be knit together and held in place with increasingly elaborate ritual. For as memory and predictive skills increased, so did the law of cause and effect that told people their own actions were what raised and lowered the light, kept the sky in place, held back the floods, and made the yams proliferate. The more the external mind knew about the world, the more effort was needed to maintain it. As technologies of household arts and food purification, of hunting and earliest gardening developed, people took on more complex and demanding work in every sphere. It must have seemed at times that the taboos knitting sacred human life together, with the growing multitude of deities and spirits, would collapse society under their weight. How could a woman be so many places at once? If her mate undertook a greater number of her taboos and offices in the home, who was left to tend the orchard, cut wood with appropriate mourning for the trees, dance the sun up, plant the millet, rice, or barley with the proper dances and sacrifices, plan the six-week wedding and the four-week earth renewal, lead the annual procession to the divine mountain that holds up the sky? And there were still the personal seclusions and ritual cleansings that had to be maintained.

The solution to the gathering burden of knowledge was the establishment of separate, select groups of people who would enact taboos in behalf of everyone else. Probably at first these were children of the tribal shamans and healers, expected to have as rigorous a training as their parents' in menstrual and hunting rites. Probably at first they were girls, menstruants secluded for years rather than weeks. James Frazer provides several examples that suggest this: In Dabadi, in British Papua New Guinea, "daughters of chiefs, were secluded inside raised houses for two or three years when they are about twelve or thirteen years of age, and never allowed to go down to the ground or have sunlight fall on them." [1]

Among other peoples, boys as well as girls would have been selected for a special life, a life of rigorous training and intense seclusion, to maintain the most extreme taboos for the people, to specialize in keeping certain rules of "the path" for the sake of the village as a whole. As these special groupings developed, the primary colors of their garments might have signified blood (red) and no blood (white), and words related to red, menstrual, and measure would describe them, as in English regal, royal, regalia, rule, ruler, regulations, regent, rex. Queenship, based in the word *gyne*, "woman," from *cune*, "cunt," embodied the collective power of the menstruant magnified to its greatest possible dimension. The parallel office of kingship imitated the rites of queenship; his blood was also often shed in sacrifice, and he would become a leader of the hunt (for the red fox, for example) and of other rites of bloodshed.

In some societies the royal or aristocratic—that is to say, the collective—menstruant personified the central cosmological principles. The queen, the holy mother, and the priestess were the living emissaries of deity, and deity likewise communicated through the externalized embodiment of the collective menstruant. The king and the priest, pharoah, or holy men were also living emissaries of deity. In many areas, members of menstrual elites were considered divine. Like the earlier menstruant, they could cause and prevent flood, famine, disease, and the movements of planets and seasons.

173

Though in our time, we imagine them as having absolute power and unlimited resources, extremely rigid restrictions attended the position of early kings and queens, priests and priestesses, holy men and women. They reenacted menstrual seclusion rites, often taken to an excruciating level of self-discipline, perhaps because they had to hold the world-forming principles for so much larger a population segment of "the world" than did an individual menstruant. Like her, they were often responsible for regulating light, preserving the surface of the earth, and separation of the waters. Royalty's rules were *regula*. In West Africa, among the Ewe-speaking peoples, the king was also high priest, and in former times was completely secluded from his subjects. He could only leave his dwelling at night in order to bathe and attend to bodily needs.[2]

A surviving precolumbian people, the Kogi, live on the Caribbean side of Colombia in high mountains; their priests teach non-aggressive meditative practice to the men. They honor the Mother, the sea, who is spirit and who is all memory and all possibility: "the mind inside nature," the mind of the Mother earth, who they call *aluna*. They say that in the beginning the Mother bled and she was fertile, and so the world was fertile, and that blood and water are what is necessary for life. Their sun priests—called "Mamas"—are selected by divination and secluded at birth in the dark, sometimes in a cave, to spend their time meditating on the Mother, the world outside only an idea taught by the older priests until the moment of their emergence into light after nine years—even as long as thirty years—of darkness. During this time the sun priest initiates ate no meat, no salt, and drank only lukewarm water, proscriptions honored for millennia by menstruants around the world.[3] Water, as well as light, taboos can be found in the royal traditions of a number of cultures. The ruler of the Ewe-speaking people of West Africa could not look upon the sea, and for this reason he was never allowed to leave his capital.[4] The rulers of other West African kingdoms were also prohibited from beholding the sea. Chiefs, priests, and kings were placed under prohibitions against crossing any rivers, or certain rivers, in the south of Madagascar, in Mashonaland (Zimbawbe), in Senegal, and also in ancient Ireland, especially on certain days.[5]

Royalty could not touch themselves, nor could ordinary folk touch them, as is still true of the queen of England today; Princess Diana was considered radical for breaking the taboo in the 1980s by shaking hands without wearing gloves. The traditions that grew up around royal menstrual taboos created the absolute formality and self-control of the traditional aristocracy. They often had to be fed and dressed by others all their lives; their hair and nails had to be especially protected so no one could steal them for magical purposes and do harm. Every substance of their bodies was imbued with extreme power; every part of their bodies had significance. A class of attendants developed around them for the primary purpose of caring for their dangerous, life-sustaining bodies: hairdressers, cosmeticians, tailors, body servants, handmaidens, kingsmen, emissaries, spokesmen, ladies of the bedchamber.

Like menstruants, royalty in many cultures could not touch the ground. They were carried everywhere on the shoulders of special servants, just as menstruants had once been carried on their grandmother's shoulders:

> Formerly neither the kings of Uganda, nor their mothers, nor their queens might walk on foot outside the spacious enclosures in which they lived. Whenever they went forth they were carried on the shoulders of men of the Buffalo clan, several of whom accompanied any of these royal personages on a journey and took it in turn to bear the burden. The king sat astride the bearer's neck with a leg over each shoulder and his feet tucked under the bearer's arms. When one of these royal carriers grew tired he shot the king onto the shoulders of a second man without allowing the royal feet to touch the ground.[6]

In other cultures, royalty would be carried in litters and divan chairs, completely covered so no one could see them—just as menstruants were carried in covered sledges on the North American continent, and as brides of north Africa went home from their weddings completely draped from head to foot, in tents atop their camels, unseen by strangers.[7]

175

The men of the royal class also inherited the menstrual and birthing thrones, the shoes, gloves, hats and long capes, and the bridal divans of women. The footwear of royalty provided ritual protection for both king and people: "According to ancient Brahmanic ritual a king at his inauguration trod on a tiger's skin and a golden plate; he was shod with shoes of boar's skin, and so long as he lived thereafter he might not stand on the earth with his bare feet." [8] The holy man of the Dogon is required to wear sandals, for otherwise his feet will burn the earth; the sandals cool him. In his sandals, he impersonates the sun, which for the Dogon is in the female domain. Among other restrictions, he is not allowed to sweat, and no one is allowed to touch him. [9]

Style of dressing, of movement, and of gesture would form the bodies of royal and holy persons just as it did those of women in general. The royal hands, like the hands of menstruants, were particularly dangerous, so they could not touch themselves or do ordinary work. Consequently, their gestures became very controlled, turned slightly outward, away from the body, in what came to be called "elegance," "delicacy," and "refinement"—and also, and of course historically accurately, "effeminate."

The menstrual chair of the tribal and village woman became the throne of royal and priestly persons. The special furniture of the menstruant passed into the royal office, too: "Among the Bakuba, or rather Bushongo, a nation in the southern region of the Congo, down to a few years ago persons of the royal blood were forbidden to touch the ground; they must sit on a hide, a chair, or the back of a slave, who crouched on hands and feet; their feet rested on the feet of others. When they traveled they were carried on the backs of men; but the king journeyed in a litter supported on shafts." [10] Among some peoples, the king was sacrificed in ancient times, and his blood might have been sprinkled upon the throne in a manner imitative of menstruation. Kings cheated, after a while, using substitutes for the sacrifice. The royal stool's relation to menstruation and crossover use in parallel menstruation is evident in an example from early twentieth-century Angola, in which the court literally bathed in the blood of a stand-in for the king:

> On the day of the ceremony the king takes his seat on a perforated iron stool, his chiefs, councillors, and the rest of the people forming a great circle round him. . . . The victim is then introduced and placed in front of the king, but with his back towards him. Armed with a scimitar the king then cuts open the man's back, extracts his heart, and having taken a bite out of it, spits it out and gives it to be burned. The councillors meantime hold the victim's body so that the blood from the wound spouts against the king's breast and belly, and, pouring through the hole in the iron stool, is collected by the chiefs in their hands, who rub their breasts and beards with it, while they shout, 'Great is the king and the rites of the state!'[11]

Similar customs are believed to have been practiced by early European royalty as well and may have been part of Celtic skull worship, the skull (of King Bran, for example) being obtained from the living king, who offered it to his suffering soldiers to use for prophecy after decapitation.[12]

The chairs of the Sumerian goddess Inanna were anointed with blood. One hymn to Inanna describes a procession in her honor: "The priest, who covers his sword with blood, sprinkles blood,/He sprinkles blood over the throne of the court chamber."[13] In miniature shrines at an ancient Cucuteni site, in present-day Moldavia, a chair of sacred significance was found, along with an altar and round oven. The chair, on which in all menstrual logic a goddess statue would have been placed during the dark of the moon, had decorative horn shapes on the back. Other miniature terracotta thrones, with large round cut-outs in the center, have been found in a Balkan site dating from the fifth millennium B.C.E.[14] One fat goddess figure from the Central Anatolian Neolithic period is seated, giving birth, chair flanked by two female lions, whose tails loop up over her shoulders. The lions are metaforms, not of her "protection of animals," as has been suggested, but of the predatory creator, the bloody-mouthed correlative of the jackal, or the

177

black leopard of menstrual origin.[15] The collective menstruant sits controlled in her chair, but her lion of death sits with her, for the danger inherent in menstrual consciousness never leaves us.

We know now what a chair is: a chair is a container for menstrual power and a conveyance of menstrual creation authority. The Greek word for menstruation is *katamenia,* "the moon below," and for chair *katahedra,* "the seat below"—hence *cathedra,* "bishop's chair"—which came to be kept in a "cathedral." Even today, a university position or a judgeship is a "chair," and the head of a corporation is its chairman, or chairperson. In England at one time a newly elected member of Parliament might be carried in triumph in a chair.[16] The proper seating of royalty and deity was on the throne, and this scene of authority *seated in place* would have given subject populations a greater sense of security and well-being than almost anything else. The most respected gods, emperors, and holy figures worldwide would be those who sat on thrones, whether "in heaven" or on earth. The throne itself sometimes acquired the divinatory power of seated authority; passages in the Bible (Revelations 16:17 and 19:5) describe a speaking throne.

The *cosmetikos* of aristocracy and royalty would also have led to the idea of accumulated riches. "Rich" is another of those words of *r'tu.* Rich is related to color, especially red; the deeper and redder the color, the "richer" it is considered to be. Richness is a form of *cosmetikos,* and the more *cosmetikos* the queen and king wore, the more protected the people felt from the powers of destruction. So royalty was draped in rubies, amber, and other metaformic stones and metals. Their coffers were filled with excess jewelry, and their bodies and thrones were cushioned with deep reds, oranges, and purples. Red carpets were rolled out for their meticulously shod feet, and parasols and canopies were held over them to shield their heads from light. Their places of abode, and often of severe restriction, were draped with the rich *cosmetikos* as well—the walls, floor, ceilings, the outsides of the buildings. The staff attending them, and the animals on which they rode (to be "off the earth")—elephants, oxen, camels, horses—they, too, were draped with *cosmetikos.*

The Goddess as Collective Menstruant

The royal and priestly menstrual elites of the world were known into historical times as "divinities." It seems reasonable to suppose, then, that the prototype for their offices and rites was the central *r'tu* of the menstruant, which initiated and guided our comprehension of divinity. I consider deity, particularly "the goddess," any goddess, as the menstruant externalized in metaform, and synchronized with elements of wilderness, *cosmetikos,* and the narrative (or path) of the menstruant.

Being always within the metaformic equation, the menstruant was a version of "the goddess" whenever she was thought to embody the earth and its elements. In seclusion rites, her skin is "the same as" the earth's surface; her bones are the same as sticks; her hair is the same as flowing water or trees and plants; her moisture is the same as rain, dew, well water, lake water, the sea. Her placenta is the same as the ground; her vulva is the same as the red ant mound. The menstruant's blood is the same as animal meat and animal blood, and both are the same as the red hot embers of the fire.

Conversely, natural formations on the earth have been equated with parts of a woman's body: a chasm or cave whose vaginal shape made it sacred to local people; breast-shaped mountains, such as the "Paps of Anu" in Ireland; the delta areas where freshwater rivers run into the ocean were especially sacred to goddesses, for instance, Oshun of West Africa. The waters of the Tigris and Euphrates were said to have streamed from Tiamat's eyes. Ideas of divinity and *cosmetikos* seem to have worked back and forth between humanity and nature, as the elements came to be comprehended in menstrual terms, and conversely, as the menstruant embodied natural principles. At times the earth was dressed as a woman: at some very ancient locations caves were smeared with

179

red ochre as though their outside edges were the lips of a menstruating or birthing vulva. At times the woman was dressed as the
earth, for example, when she cut the four directions into her flesh
or cut her daughter's hair squarely at the forehead to signify the
four directions, or when seeds or gems were embedded under her
skin as they were also planted in the earth's flesh.[17]

Menstruants dressed themselves as trees, wrapping green boughs
about their bodies and heads as protective garb. Trees might also
be dressed as a woman. In Russian villages, a birch tree was cut,
dressed as a woman, and thrown into the river on the third day of
what surely was a goddess ceremony, the tree perhaps serving as
substitute for earlier sacrificial menstruants.[18] The goddess Hera of
early Greek religions was cared for by her priestesses in the form
of a plain slab of oak about forty inches high. Later, a slab of wood
was carved in the shape of a woman and became Hera's statue—
both tree and menstruant. Later still, Hera's "image" was worked
in stone.[19] Asherah, an early Hebrew goddess, took the form of a
tree, as did the goddess Helen on the island of Rhodes, and Yggdrasil, the World Tree of Nordic myth, whose roots penetrated to
the underworld. The spirits of creation, the deities, that were defined by the collective powers of blood and by wilderness metaforms were encompassed by male rites as well. The divine principle, to which men entrained in parallel menstrual rites, was both
male and female: Snake was sometimes a goddess, sometimes a god.

In trying to comprehend the central cosmological metaform expressed as an external creator, a goddess, I think again of the earth
mother of the Dogon people, with her red ant mound vulva and
her desirable sexual relationship with the sky god's rain and her
undesirable sexual relationship with the jackal of death. When the
people laid the red fiber skirt on the ant mound, the earth goddess
was being dressed, just as the Dogon menstruant was presumably
at one time dressed. It seems completely likely that goddess images,
whether drawn on cave walls, pressed into clay, or carved in wood
or stone, were icons of a figure that had existed since the first human consciousness: the menstruant in her mask of *cosmetikos*, im-

180

personating the metaforms of cosmological consciousness, enacting the cycles to which her blood entrained her.

Impersonating Birds and Other Emissaries of Light

In her analysis of the woman-centered religion of ancient Europe, Marija Gimbutas has examined hundreds of clay figures from the Black Sea area, some nearly thirty thousand years old. These female figures are ceremonially dressed, painted, and scored. Some are seated on chairs or stools, and many wear earrings and others *cosmetikos*. Sometimes they incorporate primary wilderness metaforms: snake-headed figures, and others that wear caps and dresses and tenderly hold long vaginal snakes with discernible lips, whose bodies twine up from between the women's skirted legs.[20] These clay goddesses seem to clasp the original "Female Instructing Principle" of synchroneity.

Bird forms are also included in these goddess figures, human and female from the neck down, but with a bird's head, the noselike beak accentuated. Little dovelike birds of clay were found with the fat goddess figurines seated in the miniature shrines of the Cucuteni culture. Many other goddesses, both in mythology and archaeology, are closely connected to creatures, but only to certain creatures, repeatedly portrayed—metaformic creatures.

It seems to me that for early peoples metaformic creatures, because of a particular shape, color, or habit, embodied a theological idea or spirit. When people "shaped themselves" to that creature, they were honoring and displaying their own mental principle of what organized and shaped their universe. Even today, many peoples venerate particular animals as ancestors.

The Snake we know as synchronous flow and cyclicity from its use in origin stories and menstrual stories. The meanings of birds and the reason for bird goddesses are also suggested in origin stories, and in *cosmetikos*. Birds wake at dawn, and so they are harbingers of light; birds who make the most noise at dawn became especially metaformic and were incorporated into human culture.

Their colors added to their significance. Both prairie chickens and turkeys, revered and imitated among the peoples of the North American continent, display prominent red, purple, and orange coloring. In Malaysia and India, cocks were bred solely for ceremonial purposes as fighters; they were released into a ring in order to draw blood from each other with their crescent spikes. They were bred not only for broad breasts and strength, but also for black feathers, black skins, and black bones, which gave them magic and medicinal value.[21] Other cultures used red, white, and black roosters and chickens for blood sacrifice. In one African folktale, the rooster crows at dawn, marking the red light as the first light and thus "creating" it. Three crows of the cock also signifies death, and betrayal, as we know from Christian myth. In Asian mythology, the red rooster is associated with the underworld.

The most frequent birds in origin stories are white, however. Since the moon is also white and moves across the sky, white birds served a very special function in helping the human mind to "see" and understand the moon as a single entity. Birds also helped to "raise the sky" and to draw attention to its dimensionality. The white birds that land on the surface of reflective water and then fly up into the sky helped to differentiate the "water below from the water above," to explain how the moon could be seen in a lake and also in the sky.

The bird appears in mythology as a main character in the distinction between sky and land, and also between water and land. White birds appears in creation mythology, especially the water birds that resemble the full moon in their bodies and the crescent in their necks. These include the swan, crane, stork, and white goose. In East African myth, it was said "that once the moon was much closer to earth so that she looked like a lovely white bird."[22]

The flight of large white birds helped teach spatial relationships and perception of the moon as an entity in and of itself, rather than say, a hole in the canopy of sky. One interpretation of the Babylonian hero Marduk, who split Tiamat in half to form the world, is that he was a white dove.[23] Perhaps the white dove signified the

182

moon or particular star in this story, and people learned from following the movements of birds how to separate the sky from the earth and further their knowledge of orientation and the shape of the universe. The biblical flood, as well as other Flood stories, ends with a white dove sent out from Noah's ark, of which the *third* flight is successful in finding, that is, in re-creating, dry land. In the ancient Hebrew tradition, following instructions specified in Leviticus, at the end of seven days of menstrual seclusion the woman bathed in a special pool and took white doves to the temple for sacrifice, in payment of the blood debt of consciousness.[24]

Water birds are particularly associated with creation of the solidity of the earth's surface. They play a special part in many myths of North and South America, in which only water exists at first, and only later is the land built up out of clay or mud brought up by the birds from the bottom of the sea or lake. In an Iroquois creation myth, water birds break the fall of Sky Woman, who slips through a "hole in the sky" down into this world, which is made only of water. Sky Woman, who is also known as Falling Woman, holds a tree whose flowers are light. Turtle arrives in time for the birds to pile mud on its back, forming solid earth. Interestingly, before catching Sky Woman, some of the water birds see her as arising from below, others as falling from above. She is like the moon, sometimes mirrored in the waters of the earth, as the moon is in ponds, rivers, and lakes, sometimes in the sky.

Birds have been a major part of *cosmetikos*, not only because we have worn their feathers, but because entire cultures have built dances, songs, garments, and stories around the activities of significant birds. In some cultures, people have gone to spectacular lengths to form their bodies into the bodies of birds, surely a practice arising from the need to display metaformic ideas. The broad beaks of water birds were imitated on women's faces in parts of Africa: "Vast wedge-shaped or circular lip plates are worn by the Kichepo of south-east Sudan. They have long been considered an essential part of a woman's adornment and were traditionally worn in the presence of men or mothers-in-law." The women "extend their lips to make themselves look like certain birds—broadbills and spoonbills, for example."[25]

In ancient Europe, the large, sharp nose was revered as a beak; many clay figurines of the old goddess religion feature bird faces—sharp protruding noses, large eyes, small chin, thin mouth and striped markings. These "bird goddesses" were kept in shrines and placed on altars. It seems reasonable to imagine that women in these ancient cultures set standards of beauty based in bird features and formulated menarchal rites equating themselves with birds.

Standards of beauty and desirability based in bird qualities have continued into recent times. The Romans considered a strong beaked nose to be a sign of strong character. In northern Europe, a long pale neck was a standard of beauty, after the swan; modern American advertisements for perfume and other beauty products often still associate a woman's resemblance, or desired resemblance, to the swan. Women on a restricted diet will be described as "eating like a bird," and in England, a slang word for a desirable woman is "bird."

The recurrent image of the water bird in *cosmetikos* and in myth may reflect the ancient need to enact the ideology of the separation of the waters as part of the creation story, and to that end to help the moon take on its own independent character. The moon was no longer simply a reflection or spirit moving in the waters of the earth and sky, but a body with its own nature, free moving in its own course, like a large white bird.

Icons and Images:
The Fat Red Moon Goddess in the Fitted Cap

The earliest goddess figurines stress the roundness of the female form—of the head, breasts, hips, and stomach—to such an extreme that the concept "round" itself is expressed. These figures were at one time identified as "Venuses" and later as "Earth Goddesses." They were called "Venus" because they are naked and because their arms are diminished like the ancient Greek Statue "Venus de Milo" whose arms were broken off; they were related to "Earth" because of the heaviness of their bodies, with emphasis on breasts and belly. But we must remember that it is only relatively recently that the earth has been understood as round and imagined as a globe. For the last few thousand years most peoples portrayed the earth as a strip between the sky and the belowworld, as a floating island (Turtle), or as a square or rectangle with four directions or four legs. We must therefore pursue the goddess figures deeper into the ritual past.

The familiar fat goddess known as "The Venus of Willendorf," a stone statuette some thirty thousand years old, is about four and a half inches high and of a light red coloration. She has huge and emphatic round breasts, a round stomach, and round hips drooping over her large thighs. Her arms are prehensile, lacking muscle or bone, and are looped over her breasts. Her head is large and round, and bowed. She wears a close-fitting cap pulled down over her eyes and face; it is plaited, or perhaps knotted, in circular rows. In short, she fits the description of a royal menstruant selected to stay in seclusion for years without moving. She has become as fat and round as humanly possible. Emerging pale and moonlike from her menarchal seclusion, she is painted red. Her fitted cap protects the light, the landscape, and the people from the dangerous glance of her eyes. It comes completely down over her face so that her mouth is also safely covered, and she, having created speech, is silent so as not to misuse it.[26]

The goddess of Willendorf exemplifies the full moon metaform, the sculptural version of the Mystery. She has been identified as pregnant, and that is indeed probably one of the meanings of her shape. But to me she does not look so much pregnant as extremely fat, with emphasis put on her overall roundness, especially in her breasts and buttocks. There is no angularity in her, and her arms are tiny, expressionless, and still, resting on top of her voluminous breasts. Except for her cap and a bracelet—the navel string—she is naked, her head bowed in typical menstruant posture. Similar

185

figures have been found across southern and eastern Europe and in North Africa.[27] While many of these figures don't wear sculpted hats, and some of them are apparently pregnant, they all have their heads lowered in the posture characteristic of the menstruant emerging from her hut. Moreover, they have no faces, especially no mouths or eyes. Their legs are held tightly together, and their hands and arms are either prehensile loops or nonexistent—no chance that they will scratch their bodies.

In various sites, the figures were often found in little compartments under the floor, with flat stones enclosing them, as though they had been placed there in seclusion to protect the household. These goddess figures thus may be seen as the collective menstruant, and all that she embodied of cosmology and *cosmetikos*. "Goddess" is indeed the correct title, for they captured the central embodiment of divine protection and creation. These icons were just as metaformic in their statement as Rainbow Snake, Coyote, earth's vulval red ant mound, or Red Eel Woman—menstrual deities based in wilderness powers. Goddess icons were the *cosmetikos* of the collective menstruant translated into craft materials: clay, stone, and wood.

The goddesses of ancient Greece also displayed the characteristics of flesh and blood menstruants: Medusa, her hair writhing with vaginal snakes, had an ability that was also imputed to menstruants in some cultures: she turned living things to stone with her gaze. She is the menstruant naked, out of control, without protective *cosmetikos*. Gaia, the earth, was a chasm guarded by a great python. Long-tressed Demeter was also the earth, and her daughter Kore, or Persephone, the maiden, was portrayed holding the menstrual pomegranate. Kore disappeared and her mother went to look for her—a common menarchal drama for some peoples. Hera was "the bride," dressed austerely in long gowns. Hecate was the dark moon, portrayed as an old woman. At Sumer, alabaster statues of the large-eyed moon goddess Ningal were dressed, fed, and washed; even the urbane goddess Inanna was portrayed in one statuette holding a scratching stick, adorned with the *cosmetikos* of a temple courtesan.

186

Frequently ancient figurines portray two women together, sometimes melded like Siamese twins, side by side. Often these "dolls" wear skirts, eye and lip makeup, and hoop earrings. Frequently they are stained red. Similar dolls are still made for girls to play with in North Africa, India, and parts of the Middle East. Some of the modern dolls are of a man and woman side by side. My guess is that the paired icons were originally two sisters, representing synchronous flow. The dolls, I was told vehemently by the import shop clerk, have nothing to do with lesbianism, and I'm certain that in any current patriarchal religious system, that is true. But in more female-centered older societies, the Andean, for example, and in many parts of Western society, homosexual relations have a rightful, appropriate, and even sacred place. It thus seems significant that in the south of India, among goddess-worshiping Tamils of the Untouchable caste, a name for lesbian lover is "sister-sister."

Many goddess mythologies feature two creation sisters. Pele, the Hawaiian volcanic fire goddess who creates the earth's surface, has a sister who is "Sea Mist." Among the Pueblos, sister goddesses Naotsete and Uretsete create objects under a blanket they hold between them.[28] Sometimes one sister dwells in the world below, "in the shade," the place of the dark moon, while the other rules above, as with Egyptian Isis and her underworld sister Nepthys. The oldest known menstrual narrative of the meetings of two such sisters is the Sumerian poem, "The Descent of Inanna to the Underworld," whose metaformic meanings I will decipher later. A Caribbean proverb summarizes an ancient attitude of female "flow": "When a woman loves another woman, it is the blood of the Mother speaking."[29]

Goddesses of the Moon's Phases

Once the crescent shape was clearly identified, the moon's phases could be fixed at four: dark, full, and the two crescents. These shapes are still central to the designation of the moon's quarters. In India, each of four major Hindu goddesses is completely equated with a particular phase of the moon and with an aspect of the

187

menstrual cycle. According to Nik Douglas and Penny Slinger, authors of *Sexual Secrets,*

> the cycle of woman is compared to that of the moon, which changes and creates different influences at the different periods, ultimately returning to its original status. In the Tantric tradition a woman is viewed as a virgin (Kumari) just after menstruation, as a young wife (Saraswati) during the week following menstruation, as a worldly mistress of the house (Lakshmi) during the next week, and as a wise lady (Kali) during the approach to menstruation. During menstruation itself she is "beyond worldliness," "dead to the world and its responsibilities," and therefore freed from household duties. It is during this time that she serves as a link between this world and the next.[30]

These four names define the phases of the moon as a complex life cycle. Each of the names—Kumari, Sarasvatī, Lakṣmī, and Kali—identifies an individual goddess, but at the same time each is part of the whole. They are "aspects" of the great mystery of moon and blood that gave us the ability to name "the goddess" in the first place. Specific metaforms have accrued to each goddess pertaining to her particular place in the life cycle, and believers devote themselves primarily or exclusively to one goddess, one aspect of menstrual arts.

KALI, as the dark moon, is associated with death, transformation, and blood sacrifice. Her worshipers in the past developed fierce arts and armies and have given to English such words as "assassin" and "thug," originally names of groups of her followers who in former centuries used violence to attain political ends. Nearly naked and warriorlike, she dances on the god Shiva's dead body with his intestines between her teeth, wearing a necklace of skulls—her roses. Death is not her only attribute. She was also a primal creator and giver of life, love, and compassion. She is also associated with the weaving and cloth-dying arts; calico and Calcutta are both named for her. So though she is the most destructive aspect of menstrual power, she is also its veiling. The Scottish word for young woman, "colleen," derives from Kali's name, migrating to the language of my mother's ancestral clans from India and Mesopotamia, across the channel from Europe, down from the North Sea and Scandinavia, to that part of the British Isles still called Scotia Kali.

KUMARI, the virgin, is renewal, the waxing crescent. "The view that a woman is renewed after the cessation of her menstrual period is supported by many ancient traditions. In priestly cultures the tradition is that menstruation renews virginity."[31] Having gone through the dangerous bleeding, the virgin emerges fresh, innocent, attractive, and demure.

SARASVATI is the half-moon position. She is the young wife (weef), very artful in her white dress. She is delicate, modest, and self-absorbed, an artist intellectual depicted with lute, gold ring, red book, and swan. The white swan shaped like the half moon swims up to her with a rose in its beak. She is connected to science, poetry, and the peacock, on the back of which she rides.

LAKṣMĪ is Sarasvatī's older sister, the full moon and the matron. Dressed in deep rose with a touch of red, Lakṣmī is woman in the fullness of midlife. She looks out firmly and with confidence as her cornucopia flows down her lap the gold coins of fortune. Her demeanor is stately, her *cosmetikos* rich and complex, her dress layered. Lakṣmī has a son, Ganapathy, who has a plump man's body and an intelligent face with elephant features, including a serpentine trunk. His foot rests on a stool, and on one upraised finger he holds a lingum of male sexuality. In the Indian poster of Lakṣmī, Sarasvatī, and Ganapathy that hangs on my wall, the two goddesses sit on floating lotus flowers. In the background, two white elephants stand in a shallow sea of water; they wear red blankets, and their trunks are raised in a watery coil over their crescent tusks.

In these four goddesses, the moon is completely expressed, its phases comprehended in the life cycle of every woman.[32] These goddesses combine in the person of Parvati, the Mother, who marries Shiva, the Bull, the god of creation and the male principle in whose behalf so much of female display is directed.

One of the most remarkable things about the development of deity was its ability to change or combine gender, so that male synchronicity became incorporated into the metaform at every stage of its development. The need to include the male no doubt provided the primary motive for the externalization and deification of creative comprehensions of origin as well as cause and effect relationships. At Hermione, Hera sat on a mountain named "Throne footstool," where Zeus seduced her, landing on her lap in the form of a cuckoo. Throughout his mythic history, Zeus took the form of several older wilderness metaforms, including Light, Snake, Eagle, Bull, Swan, as well as the harbinger of spring, Cuckoo.

Narrative Path of the Goddess

What we call "the goddess"—the female creative principle as she has been retained in stone, clay, and wooden images, and also in mythology and living ritual, is a compilation of compound metaformic instructions. In her portrayal in a thirty-thousand-year-old stone carving with a round featureless face, holding a crescent horn with thirteen marks, she is a cipher of time, space, number, and synchrony. In association with wilderness creatures, she expressed ideas about the world at large. In bird form, she may have brought to consciousness the distinction between the moon in the sky and the moon in water and taught the shape of the space between earth and moon. In historic times, in the lives of sacred rulers, deity expressed ideas of reincarnation and the afterlife in rituals of separation, emergence, union, and death. In sum, our metaformic structures of deity retain and help develop our ideas of the shape and size of the cosmos and the interrelationships of its elements. Probably deity—or families of deities—constitute the most all-encompassing compound metaforms the people who perform their rituals can imagine.

According to the mythologist Carl Kerényi, Hera, the "origin of all things," was from early times identified with the moon.[33] In keeping with the Greek practice of assigning a sacred number to each deity, Hera's number was three times three, nine. Her temple at Samos was a long narrow stone structure, eighteen feet across and one hundred feet long, and without light except that provided by a small door at one end. The wooden slab embodying the goddess stood in the "shade" at the other end. Her ritual included enactment of the course of the menstruant, and she was bound with lygos vines. On selected occasions, Hera disappeared from her temple "shade," and her followers, led by her priestess, searched for her. She would be found at the bank of the river Imbrasos, known for its growth of lygos, an emmenogogue. There she was unbound, washed and dressed, then carried back to her temple. Placed on a pedestal outside the door, she was the living moon "off the earth," in its light phases.

A different part of Hera's narrative metaform was enacted in Boeotia, where she (again in the shape of a wood slab) was carried to the top of a mountain in a cart pulled by oxen kept by her priestesses. There, as enactment of her "wedding" with Zeus in his form of light, she was placed in a special shed and it was set afire.[34] Hera's compound identity was thus intricately bound with trees, sacred number, seclusion and emergence, rivers, sacred plants, mountains, oxen and carts, and various kinds of light. Her narratives were called *hieroi logoi*, sacred stories. *Logos* is Greek for speech, word, and reason; *hieros logos*—sacred story—is thus Word in the Dogon sense of sacred communication, the Word that protects the womb of existence.

By identifying the menstruant's courses with the phases of the moon, early peoples were able to comprehend life as a cycle, an idea that could be applied to any number of elements: humans, animals, plants, the earth, the sky, minerals. In thus developing deity, the people entrained the menstruant's path to other forces in nature, which gave them a metaformic narrative logic that continued to expand the human mind, and the culture that embodies it, out into the wilderness.

191

Chapter 12

■■ ■ ■ ■ ■ ■ ■ ■ ■ ■ ■ ■ ■ ■ ■

Menstrual Logic in the Visible World

IN THE paradox that underlies the workings of the menstrual mind, the more knowledge of the earth and its marvelous but unforgiving laws surfaced in human consciousness and metaformic language, the more fearful, controlling, and rite-driven humans must have become. The better we became at recalling past disasters and fearing future ones, the more often sacrifice became a major part of our actions of insurance and appeasement, and the more certain we were that the deities and spirits needed to be fed or "paid" blood, blood, and more blood.

It is easy enough to imagine how cause and effect became entangled, creating sacrificial murder. Of all the ancestral women bathing in the river at the end of their periods—whether slapping their thighs and exulting or bowing their heads to prevent harm—once in a while one would have slipped and drowned. Must that not mean the river is hungry for women? So why not go the next step and feed a menstruant to the water, or to the "Snake" of the water—especially if times were hard—as a thanks offering or a prayer for plentiful food or to prevent flood.

Tribal accounts of blood sacrifice make it clear that the killer-shaman-priest identified with the victim, who was feeding the deity with the life force or "essence" believed to reside in blood. Evidently people in virtually every part of the globe once practiced human sacrifice of one form or another as part of the metaformic religious structure that accompanied our human development. Puberty initiates of both sexes sometimes did not survive their fumigation by smoke or their food restrictions. Virgin girls, as correlates of the new moon, were favored victims, but kings, children, young men, almost anyone, could become one of the chosen. Most cultures selected as victims those most representative of their idea of "unblemished." Mayan royal blood fed a dragon of earth energy living under the temples; Aztec hearts were offered to the sun; old blood ogresses of Africa lived in rivers and caves and ate their victims; Hawaiians placated the volcano goddess with human offerings; European grain fields soaked up sacrificial blood and left us the figures of Dracula, werewolves, and the evil mother/witch of folklore; and in Greek Dionysian rites women pursued the god in human form and tore him to shreds.

Horrible as these sacrifices may sound to us, they were not done in a spirit of cruelty; nor were the people crazed or out of control during the rite. Many of those who practiced periodic ritual human sacrifice had a reputation for gentleness in general. Farming cultures, in particular, must have felt the need to feed the earth, crop, and rain deities on blood, lest they disrupt the delicate and complex cycle of growth and wipe out their entire people with famine. People thought of blood as payment due to powerful deities, who as we have seen, were metaformic to begin with. It might be said that people were, with sacrifice, "menstruating" publicly for the benefit of the forces of creation. Throughout the development of culture we have remained, like the oldest ancestress, only one step ahead of the jackal, who lives in our psyches.

Sacrifice and Compassion (1)

The summer I turn twelve years old, I suddenly decide to give up my lifelong calling to be a writer and instead to become a physician. Toward this end, I bring home library books on the history of medicine, human and animal anatomy, history of the effects of

193

plagues, lives of great doctors, and so on. I make a stethoscope from a funnel and tubing, and gather bandaids and vaseline ointment into my "doctor's bag" shoebox.

Along about early August in southern New Mexico, huge banks of rainclouds gather every afternoon and release thunderous downpours that invite exuberant children to shed shoes and run screaming around the yard. The water, arriving all at one time on the hard-baked adobe earth, tears down from the nearby mountains in deep arroyos, washing out certain north-south roads and leaving schoolyards and ball fields under a foot of standing water that takes as long as two or three weeks to disappear. During this time an inquisitive child can, by squatting in the mud and peering closely into the puddles, daily follow the remarkable transformations of the tadpoles, from their big-headed fish-shapes to the budding of legs and finally their emergence as golden-eyed toads, which grow quite large and fat and hide in reedy ditch banks.

By summer's end, I am bored with bandaging my dog and the neighbor children. My attention is caught by descriptions and illustrations in the anatomy book of the insides of humans and other creatures. I cannot get enough of the fine colored drawings of muscles and nerves, bones and veins, with thin lines out to Latin names: fibula, gluteus maximus, and vena cava. I copy some of them, pretending I am in medical school. One of the illustrations is of the inside of a frog, and I stare at it for a long time, with growing excitement. I could do that, I think.

Menstruation of the Sun and Moon

The religion of Hera included, besides the *hieros logos* that replicated the menstruant's course, special games, which Carl Kerényi believes originated what became the Olympic games. Among many peoples, not only the menstrual "race" but more elaborate games that embodied understandings of the workings of the cosmos evolved as part of menstrual *logos*, logic that begins with story. Story was thus the verbal expression of what had earlier been ritual enactments. Just as the menstruant impersonated the moon, protomoon, or sun in her seclusion, so too did the sacrificial victim of sun or moon rites, as public menstruant. Evidently ball games also became a method of involving the entire community in learning the movements of the sun and moon and connecting them to their own survival.

"Of all the ball games that were being played in North, Central, and South America at the time of European contact, the Mesoamerican game, which used a rubber ball and was played on masonry ball courts, was the most elaborate. In the Mesoamerican game, players were divided into two teams which faced each other across the center of the court. These players *could not touch the rubber ball with their hands,* so they wore heavy padding of leather, wood, and woven materials over the places where they could strike the ball, their hips and knees."[1] Players tried to hit the ball, either through the opponents' end zone or through a ring tenoned into the side wall. That the players could not touch the ball with their hands is completely congruent with the special protections and restrictions surrounding the hands of the menstruant and the prohibitions against touching her own blood, for the balls in this game were equated to blood. According to the Popol Vuh, the sacred text of the Quiche Maya, one part of the ball game series was played on the summer solstice, when the sun and moon were believed to mate in order to conceive the maize. The moon goddess was Xquic, a name that also meant "rubber" and "blood."

Rubber was probably at one time blood also for certain people of the Amazon River area, who coat boys with rubber and then cover them with downy white feathers as part of their puberty ceremony. Rubber is a particularly interesting metaform in that it can be formed into a round object that bounces—returning along the course of its projection. Hence it could in several ways be equated with the shape and movements of the moon or sun, still retaining its quality as the "blood" of the tree, analogous of course to the blood of women. It seems reasonable to suppose that the reason Mayan ball players were thickly muffled in gloves, helmets, and other padding and could not touch the rubber ball is that the ball was metaformically "the same as" menstrual blood.

The Popol Vuh, which narrates the elaborate ball game myth, makes it clear that the game was not a simple sport but an annual or semiannual rite of world formation. In the myth the belowworld powers, the lords of Xibalba who rule the realm of death, both vanquish and renew the lords of light: "This ball game played on the vernal equinox would probably culminate with the sacrifice of a player chosen to represent the descending sun. The sacrifice of this player would cause the descent of the sun by sympathetic magic, for the sun is also sacrificed when he descends into the underworld."[2] The ball game played on the autumnal equinox, conversely, ended with the sacrifice of a player who represented the moon goddess, whose death heralded the return of the sun. Thus the sun and moon both bleed as they go into underworld seclusion. To this basic narrative were also connected the summoning of rain and the mating of sun and moon to produce the corn that was the economic foundation of the Mayan culture.

The sun maize is born in the autumn during the corn rites of first fruit; the moon goddess dies giving birth and is instantly reborn, to take her place in the sky. Temple observatories established precise dates for these events, and some of the names of the deities are also dates in the Mayan calendar. Horizontal space was divided into the four directions, with a fifth at center. Vertical space was imagined in the three layers, sky, earth, and belowworld. In the ball court myth, the earth was imagined as a narrow strip with eastern and western ends. The western end, which swallows the sun or moon, was a jaguar, which as we know was the Mesoamerican version of Wolf, Jackal, Fox, Dog, and Coyote of other mythologies. The eastern end, which spews forth the renewed sun and moon, was—why are we not surprised?—a serpent with open mouth.

In this series of ball games a lunar/menstrual logic was at work, equating the movements of the sun—and also, some authorities on Mayan culture think, Venus—with the lunar/human cycles of blood, birth, and death. The unity of cosmogony, economy, and

196

spirituality was displayed in one whole enacted thought. The Mayan ball game is an example of how human beings absorbed astronomical observations into the life-and-death mythos of the people. The game was not played for entertainment or to display athletic prowess and courage, though of course it did both. The ball game was a religious rite that also enacted scientific principles with human players, whose real deaths imprinted the lesson as perhaps, at the time, nothing else could have.

Sacrifice and Compassion (2)

I have no trouble acquiring the necessary tools for my dissection. My father has recently given me an exacto kit, so I have sharp blades. My mother's bathroom cupboard yields a bottle of rubbing alcohol and some cotton, and the neighborhood pharmacist matter of factly sells me a small can of ether.

One single turn about the yard of our apartment easily brings a young, light green, gold-eyed toad leaping into my young hands, and from there into a coffee can, until I have made my preparations. As I lay out the knives and the cotton on a white dishtowel, wiping the blades with alcohol, I have the distinct feeling of changing from one kind of person into another. The ether-soaked cotton affects the toad at once, and as I turn the unconscious body over onto the clean white dishtowel, I feel important, logical and clinical, extremely self-controlled. I study the anatomy illustration to make my cuts in the thick, cream-white skin, skin the texture of soft, well-cared for leather.

I marvel at the amount of glistening life held within her bag of skin, amazed at how beautiful the organs are. Far more vivid than the illustrations, they glisten with life and color. The startling beating heart in particular draws my attention, then the tender lungs and membranes, and the sudden surprise of dozens of blue-black eggs richly clustered in her abdomen. For ten minutes or so, I breathe my wonder at her pulsing life force. I have fallen in love with her.

197

Then comes the eye of truth. Her heart is steadily beating; her whole body is vulnerable before me; my "doctor experience" with the miracle of life is completed—and now what? Nothing in the anatomy texts tell me how to sew her up again. There are no adults around for me to ask; no other children would know the answer either. I am alone with her.

With growing horror, I realize I have to kill her. That I have already killed her. That, by not taking her whole life into account, in choosing to look so far inside her, I chose also to kill her. I realize her eggs will never be born.

I lean over her with the knife tip aiming at her beautiful heart, my own heart breaking with understanding. "I'm sorry," I whisper repeatedly, knowing I will never again trust simple curiosity, knowing too that medicine, making whole, is based in a multitude of cuttings, and deaths. I bury her, throw away the cotton and the dishtowel, tell no one what I have done. I had thought the dissection of the toad would further my knowledge of anatomy and of healing. Instead, it teaches me compassion for "small" lives and deepest shame, the certain knowledge of my ability to do irreparable harm even in the name of doing good. And the gift she gives me is remorse.

Menstruation of the Sky

As human cultures developed, menstrual logic, the stories we tell about the world, fanned out in ever extending arcs. Or rather, I could say that human development was created by the extension out from the hut of menstrual logic, the *logos* entraining with ever larger visible cycles of nature. Not only the sun and moon, but other celestial figures that follow the east-west course, were swept into the expanding menstrual mind, which provided the "plot" for comprehending natural phenomena and for connecting them to human activities.

The constellation called the Seven Sisters, or Pleiades, was one of the features of the sky that thus became incorporated into metaformic logic. Many peoples connected the little squarish cluster of stars to blood sacrifice and cutting:

> The sacrifice of the Mexican savior Xipe Totec, our Lord the Flayed One, took place on the Hill of the Stars at the moment when the Pleiades reached the zenith on the last night of the Great Year cycle. . . . In ancient India the Pleiades were called the Seven Mothers of the World, or Krittikas, "razors" or "cutters." . . . The Pleiades were prominent in the early cult of Aphrodite, who was supposed to have given birth to them under her name of Pleione. Aphrodite was a castrating Crone-goddess as well as a Holy Dove; and the Pleiades were "a flock of doves." They were connected with sacrificial New Year ceremonies in Greece as in central America and southeastern Asia. The Seven Sisters stood at the zenith on New Year's Eve as if to select the god of the new Aeon. Old Babylonian texts began the year with the Pleiades.[3]

They are "emanations" of the moon goddess in classical mythology and thus are also menstrual blood. That they are so frequently referred to as seven sisters implies that they embodied synchronous flow, associated with blood, sacrifice, and significant times of the year. These associations are explicitly in a myth of the Barasana people of Columbia. The Barasana identify Opossum with the Pleiades, which sets in the west just as the long South American dry season ends and the rainy season begins.[4]

In the myth, the woman Yawira has an appointment with Tinamou Chief. Along the way she is tricked by Opossum into meeting him instead, and she goes to live with the foul-smelling creature for a while. One day she disobeys Opossum's warning not to look downstream, and she sees Tinamou Chief. She goes to him, though he initially rejects her because she has acquired a bad smell from Opossum. Then Opossum and Tinamou quarrel, and Opossum is killed, and at that moment the rains begin.

Tinamou Chief is the Sun, the tinamou being a yellow bird. Opossum is, as we know, a metaform for the moon. In the web of connections between this story and shamanic rite for the Barasana, the woman Yawira is also a form of the mother of the sky, Romi

Kumu, who is represented in their ritual as a special gourd (depicting the sky) containing beeswax. The gourd is considered a womb, and the aroma of burning wax has connotations of female sexuality. Romi Kumu is also represented by the Pleiades, whose cycle of east-west rising and setting marks a renewal of the year. The rains are considered Romi Kumu's flow of menstrual blood. "Also, in Barasana thought, the Pleiades can be the wax gourd, and the wax can be the blood. The Pleiades became the source of the rain as the gourd is the source of the wax and the vagina is the source of the blood. From the fall of the Pleiades and the death of Opossum comes renewal."[5] In the interval between dry and rainy seasons, the Barasana hold their most important ritual, at which the menstrual wax is burned, the smoke is fanned to the four directions, male and female emblems are joined to knit the year together, and certain musical instruments forbidden to the sight of women are played. This interwoven complex of metaforms, part ritual, part narrative, hold the year together, using menstrual logic to teach renewal: Opossum, like the Pleiades and the moon, brings on life-giving "menstrual" rains and never really dies.

The connective "and" relates two elements in metaphoric conjunction, sometimes giving us incremental addition—one *and* two *and* three—but also giving us our human idea of cause *and* effect. "Opossum died *and therefore* the rains began." This basis of human logic developed a multitude of variations, and gave us both dependency on emotional superstition *and* wondrous scientific control and observational skills—mixed, in every culture and era; and capable of change. For the Barasana people, the Pleiades and the mythology and ritual surrounding the constellation's periodic disappearance, or "fall," "brought" the rain, not just any rain, but predictable periodic rain, the monsoon rain necessary to establish agriculture as a human occupation and support system.

Menstruation of the Year

The Barasana myth illustrates how people made ordered use of natural events by imagining the sky as a menstruating female. They were ordering spatial events with menstrual *logos*. People also applied menstrual logic to time, especially with New Year's celebrations. For many peoples, New Year marks the confluence of at least two cycles, the solar and lunar. Presumably peoples long ago, who had not yet differentiated the two lights, would not have had a New Year. New Year, like New Moon, signified the emergence of a central character—the sun, the new moon (or both), after seclusion, perhaps followed by the "marriage" of the two principles.

New Year in ancient Mesopotamia was the most important celebration, and can be understood quite literally as the menarche of the year. Origin epics were read, priests led processions through the streets, and at Sumer the sacred marriage took place between the high (*en*) priestess and the king. Planets as well as the sun and moon were included in the sophisticated *logos* of the Sumerians. Descriptions of the menarchal and marriage preparations of the planet Venus in the person of the high priestess, and New Year's hymns to the goddess Inanna/Venus, give us a rich picture of the festivities.

The exact Sumerian New Year—the one day of the "true New Moon"—was carefully calculated by the juxtapositions of stars and planets "in order to care for the life of all the lands." On the day of the "sleeping" of the moon, a "sleeping" place was set up for Inanna as well, a bed whose rushes were cleansed with cedar oil, which must have made a satisfying red wash. This bed, cleaned of "blood," was then covered with a bridal sheet to make it safe for the king.[6]

During the seven days of the menarche-marriage, the priestess was specially washed and dressed. Her feet were washed by her *sister,* and she received gifts of clothing and jewelry, and a special dress from the king. A cake was a featured part of the festive foods, and emmer beer; wine and honey were poured for Inanna at dawn. She prepared for her lover by washing and sprinkling cedar oil on the ground. On the seventh day, the priestess and the king went to the marriage bed for a sexual consummation that is wonderfully explicit in the texts: "After he enters her holy vulva, causing the queen to rejoice/Inanna holds him to her and murmurs:/O Du-

201

muzi, you are truly my love." They did not then live together, for this coupling enacted the union of male and female metaforms, the Bull with the Morning Star, not the establishment of a new family. Any child born of the *en*-priestess was killed or put in a basket in the river. The bull god would have represented the herding economy of the countryside, as Inanna represented horticulture and the crafts of the city. They are the prototypes of Adam (Adamuzi) and Eve (Heveh, "life"). Dumuzi and Inanna had fruit trees, including an apple tree, and she was also associated with the serpent.

The New Year's procession in ancient Sumerian cities like Ur and Uruk featured the Kurgarra priests, who sprinkled blood on the throne, and an interesting array of costumed celebrants. Men and women wore the clothing of the opposite sex on half their bodies, female clothing on the left, male on the right, as if in acknowledgment of the fact that to a large extent gender roles are assigned by the menstrual mind. Young men rolled hoops and sang; male prostitutes combed their hair and wore colored scarves; young women and coiffured priestesses carried swords and double axes. Old women chose the cooks for the lavish food, wine, and beer offerings, and people competed in games with jumpropes and colored cords. Over all swelled the variety of drums and tambourines, and the dancing people were very sexual and merry.[7]

While New Moon celebrations and rites were based in the menstruation of the month, New Year celebrations and rites, sometimes including the sacred marriage, marked the menarche of the year. At Babylon on the fourth day after the "true New Year," the creation epic was read aloud, as though to re-create the world at the emergence of both the new moon crescent and the menstruant after three days of seclusion.

Like the Pleiades, the course of Venus is also in the east-west arc, and so the planet acquired the menstrual cycle and its metaformic ritual, including deification as Inanna (also called Ishtar). As the only daughter of the moon couple, Inanna inherited the whole lunar tradition.

202

Noisemaking with rattles and drums was a feature of menarchal festivities and processions, intended to frighten away the "evil spirits" of the wilderness. Stated another way, the noise reminded the people to stay alert and conscious of their surroundings. Perhaps when noisemaking acquired an orderly *cosmetikos,* music was the result. It is striking that so many musical scales are five, or as in ancient Egyptian flutes, seven notes, the standard scale played in the West. New Year's worldwide is a special time for making both noise and music, especially horned music. Men in parts of old Africa blow on antelope or other horns at the New Moon as well as New Year. In China, gunpowder was developed to fire strings of red firecrackers at the New Year, to scare evil spirits. My parents celebrated New Year's Eve by lighting candles and drinking whiskey, even my teetotaling mother at times having a special sip. At midnight my mother got an unpleasant, fearful look and covered her ears with her hands, while my father, smiling and trying all by himself to enjoy it, went out to blow a hole in the yard with his thirty-ought-six rifle, which made a fine explosion. I sat on the steps between them, drawn in both directions.

When I was in high school I went out with my friends on Halloween, which is the Celtic New Year, to soap windows as a "trick." We were too tender-hearted for more extreme pranks; but out in the countryside, young people characteristically pushed over out-buildings—sheds—and black cats hid for their lives. My mother said when she was a girl, youngsters pulled pranks such as putting a car or carriage up on a barn roof—things, reminiscent of older rites of the cosmic menstrual emergence of the New Year.[8]

Menstruation of the Earth

Given that ancient peoples drew astronomical events, periodic rainfall, the seasons, and other cycles of time and space into the net of menstrual *logos*, it is no surprise that they applied the same logical plot to the earth, viewing it as female and enacting religious rites that developed the arts of farming. A yearly menstruation of

the earth was enacted in Greece, when women separated from men
to hold the three-day fall festival Thesmophoria. They used the
emmenogogue lygos to coordinate their bleeding, and built rude
huts of its vines, replicas of the sheds of their ancestresses. The
women fasted and performed specific rites on each day, including
a sacrifice of piglets, which they carried into a deep chasm in which
lived Snake. They emerged from the earth's chasmic vulva carrying
barley seed mixed with rotting pig flesh ("menstrual" blood) for
sowing.[9]

Even into historic times people saw the dirt of the fields as
"flesh," as is suggested by the ancient Jewish custom of letting the
land "rest" from agricultural work in a Sabbath, one year in every
seven. Application of menstrual narrative logic to agricultural cycles also has had a long tradition in India, where villagers still use
menstrual terms to describe certain Hindu agricultural festivals.
According to Frédérique Marglin, in *Wives of the God King,* "the
meaning of menstrual blood can be explored [in] the festival of the
menses of the goddess, called Raja Samkranti."[10] The word *samkranti,* she explains, refers to the passage of the sun from one sign
of the zodiac to another, while menses is one meaning of *raja.* The
menses of the goddess is celebrated just before the bathing festival,
which is on the last day of June.[9]

The festival is celebrated for four days, during which time the
earth (*pruthibi*) is also believed to be menstruating. "The first day
is called First Samkranti (*pahili samkranti*); the second day is called
raja samkranti; the third day is called 'burning earth' (*bhui da-
hana*); the fourth day is called 'the bath of the Goddess' (*Thakurani
Gadua*). The 'burning earth' is so called because it is said that the
red colour of the earth at that time, due to the earth's menstruation,
makes it look as if it were on fire. This is also connected to the
belief that if one sowed any seeds during these days they would
burn up."[11]

During the four days of Raja Samkranti, the women are considered to be impure (*asauca*), as is the goddess. They do not wear
their usual vermilion mark, nor do they oil or comb their hair,

following the practices they would during their real menses. The women play, sing songs, and swing on swings made for this occasion, and their happiness is important to the rite. They are not supposed to do any domestic work, and it is the men who prepare the food during these days. The men and women abstain from sexual relations, and as a correlate to this, the men do not plow the earth. "In the words of the farmer: '*Pruthibi* is impure (*asauca*); we as human males and females we live as Isvara and Parvati, so the women observe this festival. We are Isvara and they are Parvati, so when mother goddess is impure, they, being Parvati, are also impure.'"[12]

After Raja Samkranti, the rains are expected to arrive; and when they do, the farmers again plow the earth so that the seeds can germinate: "On the fourth day of the festival, in the morning the women will bathe and the goddess in the temple will also be bathed and her body rubbed with oil and turmeric. On that day ends the prohibition to plow or to use carts for the farmers. The earth's impurity is over, and so is the women's."[13]

In keeping with the course, or plot, of menstrual *logos,* the festival that follows Raja Samkranti and the Day of Bathing, marking the end of monsoon, is the "Car Festival." The Car Festival centers around four statues, two of the sister goddesses Lakṣmī and Sarasvatī and their husband Jagannātha (Lord of the World) and his older, unmarried brother, Baḷabhadra.

For their procession, towering wooden chariots or carts are built over a two-month period before the festival. They are painted more than one color but always including red. The wood is chosen by the king, who makes the first ax stroke; the number three plays a prominent part in this rite. The beginning of the Car Festival is timed with the end of the rains; the deified images are carried out for public display, facing east. They are then vigorously washed, and taken into the temple for a "dark period" of fourteen days, in which they are considered to be in a state of illness. The statues are laid on their sides; the temple is dark and silent. The goddesses and gods may be touched only by special attendants. They are "fed"

205

only raw fruit during this time, and some medicine prescribed by the temple doctor. As the washing has smeared their paint, at the end of their lying down period, with the new moon, they are repainted. One day is set aside for the painting of their eyes. After this, the two gods and Sarasvatī are carried out to the decorated carts for a grand procession that is considered a pilgrimage by the faithful, who joyfully crowd the streets throwing fruit, coconuts, money, and jewelry into the chariots. Wooden horses are attached to the huge carts, which men drag through the street by ropes, with accompaniment of drums, bells, and songs. The three sacred figures are taken to a temple used only for the purpose of secluding them for seven days. Lakṣmī is taken separately, on a palanquin carried by priests, at night.

The procession of the gods by cart imitates the menstruant's journey. Like her the images emerge facing east. Like her they are washed. They are rubbed with oil and turmeric and repainted with *cosmetikos,* with special attention to their eyes. Thus, like her, they embody renewal.[14] The *Oxford English Dictionary* confirms that archaic meanings of "chair" included car and chariot. Related words are "carry," "carriage," and even "career," to rush down a road. From a menstrual point of view, the chair made portable is what created the covered litter, which then only needed wheels (light's shape) to become a cart. The functions of both chairs and wagons—to contain menstruants, brides, or parallel menstrual officials—remained the same for millennia. The goddess Car was prominent in Persia, not so far from the Mesopotamian area where the oldest wheeled vehicles have been unearthed by archaeologists, or from the "Car Festival" of India. The ancient place name Cardia, meaning "Car goddess," was named for her, and her name is a correlate of Q'or, Cerridwen, and Kore, the maiden daughter of the earth mother, Demeter.[15]

Variations of the original menstrual sequence became models for the great festivals of agricultural peoples, extending into every aspect of their lives. Agriculture was based in menarchal principles, establishing rules of when to plant, when to wait, when to expect rain, when to harvest, when to let the land rest. The cycles of menstruation, because they were externalized and thoroughly practiced, allowed people to trust themselves to grow their own food.

Agriculture was more than "planting by the moon." It was first and foremost modeled after the menstrual rite and the sacred wedding. Models of menstruation and sexual intercourse were applied to the earth and the sky, models of male fertility to the plowing of the ground. The menstrual mind allowed humans to spill out beyond the small gathering-hunting clan to form complex villages dependent on farming and animal husbandry of edible metaforms. To state this most succinctly, it isn't that menstrual/lunar principles and analogies were applied to farming. Rather, the externalization of increasingly complex menstrual/lunar principles are what created and developed farming. Farming grew from the application of menstrual narrative logic to certain plants, animals, the ground, and the cycles of seasons, light, and rain.

It is not surprising, then, that "plot" at once means place, area of land, burial spot, and narrative line. Nor is it surprising that, for farming peoples, blood sacrifice has seemed the best hedge against crop failure—so much of the natural world needed to be influenced by human behavior. Not only farmers but all kinds of cultures have used sacrificial murder and stories of murder, including murder of loved ones, to instruct themselves about the cycles of the world. Blood sacrifice is part of menstrual logic.

The word *r'tu*, as I have said, has three meanings: the first is *menstruation;* the second, the *special act of sexual intercourse directly following menstruation;* and the third, a *season or special time of year.* By celebrating festivals of the New Year—the menstruation and renewal of the year—humans came to understand themselves in relation to seasons and time. The New Year procession at Sumer and the great menstrual and car festivals of rural India are not so far from modern American rites—both North and South—with our New Year Rosebowl and other parades featuring decorated cars, carts, and towering images, and our New Year football games; with our Mardi Gras, Carnival, Chinese New Year

207

firecrackers and parade of dragons, and Celtic New Year masks and parades. All these celebrations mark renewals of the year and have many overlapping ancient elements—floats, costumes, statues, cross-dressing, games and sports, noise, sexual antics, flowers, and the color red. They celebrate, whether the participants remember or not, the menstrual cycle of the year.

By using the logic of metaform and the entrainment, through myth, of one cycle to another, the menstrual mind has extended out in an expanding net to encompass the movements of stellar bodies, the changing of seasons, the transitions of solstices, the greater lunar cycles, the growth of plants, and the recurrence of natural phenomena such as floods, monsoons, and volcanic eruptions. That people called these cycles "sacred" and incorporated them with ritual underscores the menstrual roots of scientific methods and classifications. In the logic of story, sometimes the sequence of rituals is told in narrative form and sometimes—as happened when I applied a textbook description to a real toad—story is reenacted in rite. As the word *logos* implies, we learned to think in storied rites, the *hieros logos,* that followed the course of the menstruant. Menstrual *logos* gave us the logical principles of thinking, our reason, which we continually revise and refine.

Chapter 13

Narratives: Descent Myths and the Great Flood

WORD migrated from *cosmetikos* to story with the development of human language.[1] Ancient narratives employed characters, plots, numbers, and orientations that had already been deeply imprinted upon human mind by millions of years of menstrual ritual. According to the Dogon philosopher Ogotemmêli, speech began as the second Word of weaving the cloth skirt, so that speaking, storytelling, spinning, and weaving all come together in myth. The spirit who wields the Dogon shuttle has a forked tongue and is thus connected to Snake. On Easter Island, if a native woman wants to tell an old story, she first makes a cat's cradle whose design "holds" the story. Word is thus *cosmetikos* spun into the air as sound.

In some cultures, the sight of another woman menstruating, or the sight of an arrow, bow, or spear might actually cause a woman to begin her period, or so the people reported. It is not surprising, then, that a story alone could also cause women to bleed. Peruvian Sharanahua women covered their ears so as not to menstruate on hearing the words of a story about Moon (a male character) causing women to bleed through sexual intercourse.[2] Remnants of the power of narrative to bring on a physical "flow" still exist in modern dramas that cause tears or sexual arousal, or in fiery speeches that succeed in persuading people to commit acts of bloodshed.

Given that story alone might have caused menstruation to begin, it is not surprising that for many peoples origin story was the same as ritual in its capacity to hold the world order together. Origin stories were incorporated into menarchal, hunting, healing, and funeral rites and were used at certain times of year to order the universe. The Kogi report that the titles of their oral origin story take nine nights to list, and the epics, nine times nine nights to tell.[3] As we know from the Babylonian rites, origin stories were associated with New Year celebrations, as they were with other seasonal menarches in the Americas.

Writing, which evidently began as *cosmetikos* with its embedded numerical, lunar, and geometric markings, was transferred to the "skin" of cloth, and then to the "flesh" of sacred pottery. Marija Gimbutas believes that the serpentine symbol painted in Magdalenian and Old European cultures in association with uterine and vulvular shapes suggests affinity between the zigzag, the letter M, and all types of female moisture. The zigzag, and its truncated form M, is the earliest symbolic motif recorded.[4] The two crescents of M perhaps also indicate it is a menstrual/lunar cipher, leading to the concurring M-words menstrual, mensural, moon, mental, measure, medium, mother, milk, moisture. The inverted M was perhaps the mother of such words as water, wicca, warrior, wagon, and of course, "word."

After thousands of years of marking symbols on pottery surfaces and divinatory plates like runic stones, flat bones, and bark tablets, our ancestors began to organize the earliest scripts. Cuneiform, beginning five thousand years ago in Sumer, was used to record grain accounts as well as religious myth. The alphabet allowed writing to be somewhat abstracted from ritual. It could then be used not only to record older stories, but also to open up new combinations of narrative that shifted from female to male origin story.

At first all written texts must have been considered sacred and surrounded with special temple ritual. Tablets from Mesopotamia found last century and translated throughout this one have given us the roots of sacred story, *hieros logos,* in the Western tradition, including the earliest written versions of the Flood myth, the creation story of Tiamat and Apsu, the creation of humans by a goddess using bits of clay, and many others. The texts of the goddess Inanna tell a nearly complete female-based drama, of her courtship and marriage, her acquisition of throne and bed, her inheritance of the sacred measurements, or laws, and of her philosophy of cycles of life and death.[5]

These earliest written myths, dated 3–2000 B.C.E. form the basis of the completely male-centered religious mythology that began to establish itself around 800 B.C.E. In particular two menstrual narratives, the Descent myth and the Flood myth, were written down in enough detail that we can trace the crossover from female to male protagonists. Just as men imitated menstruation through cutting the penis or other displays of blood during puberty rites, just as they became hunters in order to participate in blood rituals of their own, so in narrative terms they also developed central characters who imitated and replaced the original goddess metaforms.[6]

The Descent Myths as Menstrual Journeys

The Descent myth's menstrual elements are clear in texts related to the goddess Inanna/Ishtar, particularly in the poem "The Descent of Inanna to the Underworld."[7] The seclusion rites are of mythic proportions, for here Inanna is a planet, not a person: The goddess makes a voluntary journey to the underworld palace of her older sister Ereshkigal, where she is stripped, judged, flayed, and hung for three days on a peg.

To make her journey, she dresses in elaborate *cosmetikos* that display her rulership of seven of the temple-based cities of Sumer. (Inanna's temple is the oldest known, and the development of the oldest known cities should be credited to her.) These *cosmetikos,* including a crown, lapis necklace, gold ring, and decorated robe, are stripped, office by office, at each of seven gates—seven being the number of days of creation and also of menstrual seclusion in the Near East, as we know from Leviticus, a later text.

211

Once Inanna has entered the cosmic "shade" of the underworld, she is put under a silence taboo: "Silent Inanna, sacred customs must be obeyed."[8] There are food and drink taboos as well: "Even if she offers you a field of wheat, do not eat it." "Naked and bowed low" as any initiate, Inanna approaches the wooden throne of the queen of the underworld. She herself sits upon the throne, and at that moment she is pronounced "guilty." We might say that her status of menstruant is established by her action, and she then must pay the debt of consciousness with her bleeding flesh. The three days she hangs on the peg are the dark moon, and the peg itself recalls the tree wherein the moon once "hung." While Inanna bleeds on her peg, her older sister is giving birth, so the two goddesses synchronize their two kinds of bleeding, just as do the ancestral sisters of the Wawilak myth. But here death, the killing of the younger sister in the underworld, has become part of the narrative logic. The myth carefully, it seems to me, avoids blaming Ereshkigal for her sister's death. Inanna, though she is "struck" by her sister, is flayed and killed by seven "judges" of the underworld. Ereshkigal is never described as Inanna's enemy. Indeed, after the slain goddess is resurrected at the end of the myth, she says of her older sister, "Sweet are her praises."

The person who effects Inanna's emergence, and the first person she sees on her return, is Ninshubur, her "vizier," the "Queen of the East." The original menstrual principle of orientation is here personified as queen and goddess. The proscribed behavior of the gods that ultimately resurrects Inanna is also thoroughly menstrual, as is the fact that she leaves the underworld with the injunction that she must use "the Eye of Death"—consciously directing the menstrual gaze—to choose another to take her place. She will thus utter "the cry of guilt" to Dumuzi, declaring him sacrificial menstruant.

So far the story, though it contains male gods—Sky and Storm, who do not help Inanna, and Enki, god of Word and semen, who does—is a female myth of seclusion, "death" (bleeding), and regeneration. But Inanna's choice of a replacement is Dumuzi, the Bull,

212

her lover/husband, and she thus passes the role of main character in the menstrual *logos* to the male principle. In this gender shift, the story begins to change.

Dumuzi's reaction to the underworld is completely different from Inanna's. She volunteers to go and dresses grandly for the occasion; he reacts with terror and attempts several times to escape. He has himself turned into older wilderness metaforms, first a snake, then a gazelle. He goes to his mother for a dream interpretation, and to his sister's house, and to the house of an old woman, to hide from the seven demons, the *galla*, sent from the underworld to take him below by force. He begs not to go. While he is hiding among the plants of the field, the demons torture Geshtinanna, his sister, but she will not betray him. However, Dumuzi's friend (an early unnamed Judas), after promising loyalty, gives him away at the first offer of sacred grain and water. Dumuzi's stripping is violent. He is beaten, his sheepfold is torn to pieces, his bowls of milk overturned, and he is dragged into his "shade."

Yet his role as victim is still partial, for both Inanna and his mother are moved by compassion to a compromise. Dumuzi will stay in the underworld only six months of the year, and his sister Geshtinanna will serve the other half of the year in his behalf.

The underworld saga of Inanna and Dumuzi in Sumerian mythology is echoed by related stories of Ishtar and Tammuz in the neighboring Akkadian tradition; of Demeter and Persephone, Aphrodite and Adonis, Orpheus and Eurydice in the Greek; of Isis and Osiris in the Egyptian; of Nana and Balder in the Norse; of the Nisan shaman in Mongolia and the two male companions Gilgamesh and Enkidu in Babylon; and the Mayan version with the moon and sun in the Popol Vuh. The crossing of the river became incorporated into some of the versions, a river of blood, or the River Styx, or the Red River (in a Mongolian myth), or a river that must be crossed but cannot be touched.

By the time the Greeks were telling this story, Ereshkigal had been replaced by an active male principle, Hades (Pluto), and from the male point of view, Persephone's descent was an abduction. Her

213

mother Demeter, helped by the older underworld goddess Hecate, pursue her in a menstrual hide-and-seek. Women were now leaving their mothers' villages to live with their husband's kin, and the myth may have expressed the ambiguity women felt at this shift. The pomegranate is an obvious metaform, as we have seen. Persephone must not eat the rich red fruit of the dead if she wants to return to her own kinfolk. But Hades tempts her with it, and she eats the seeds. The myth makes a compromise of this wrenching situation; some of the time she lives with Hades, some with her mother. Greeks made at least one pilgrimage in their lives to Eleusis for the public reenactment of this menstrual Descent story, and the Eleusinian mysteries were the central religious rite in Greece for two thousand years. By the time the myth of Christ replaced Demeter's earth religion, the male sacrificial role was uncompromised, though the story retained the fundamental elements of the earlier female versions.

The Descent myth is the essential plot of most Western stories, featuring a crisis and a transformation. Ritual stories of war and the hunt, of ordeal and treasure-seeking, are also Descent myths. In our twentieth century accounts, emphasis has been on the crisis of sacrifice (murder, almost always featuring blood), which is forbidden. The question of who did it and why reinforces our curiosity about human psychology, our use of logic, and our ability to think in terms of cause and effect: who had motive, opportunity, and weapon? We sharpen our reasoning powers by solving little narrative mysteries that stem from the greater Mystery of our origins.

But the Descent myth is not the only menstrual story in Inanna's female lineage; she also inherited the even more widespread creation story, the Flood.

The Covenant and the Boat of Heaven

By the time written narrative developed in Mesopotamia around 3000 B.C.E., the fourth generation of Sumerian gods were well defined—the waters had divided into salty sea, land, and sky; the storm god Enlil was differentiated from Ea/Enki, the god of "sweet waters," and the moon pair had parented the sun, Utu, and his sister Inanna, the planet Venus. It is of these gods that the earliest literature of Mesopotamia tells, and the stories underlie much of the narrative-based religions of Judaism, Christianity, and Islam. Of this literature, two outstanding Flood myths survived on clay tablets through four or five thousand years of weather and human turmoil.

The evidently older of the two stories, or at any rate the most elementally tribal and direct, centers on Inanna and the god Enki. The story told in one long poem, "Inanna Meets the God of Wisdom," cannot be dated, though Inanna's statues and eight-pointed star emblem have been dated from at least 4000 B.C.E., and goddess worship that may have included her has been detected at sites twice as old.[9]

The story features a uniquely female ark, "the Boat of Heaven," a reference both to Inanna's vulva and to the crescent moon. Inanna sometimes rides a crescent moon. The Sumerian god of wisdom, Enki, known in Babylon as Ea, is the god of semen and sweet waters, and also of "the Word." In fact, he is said to be able to create because he is of "the Word." Remembering that the Dogon people recall "the Word" as the fiber skirt that marks the menstrual vulva, we can imagine that Enki/Ea is an ancient male fertility god, and directly in the menstrual/lunar lineage; in fact he is unique among male gods in that he can safely go into the underworld. He is Inanna's father-in-law in "Inanna Meets the God of Wisdom."

In the poem, the goddess, a budding young woman, leans against her apple tree and admires her own vulva, praising it out loud. Then she leaves her city to visit the city and the temple of Enki. When she arrives, his vizier (in Sumerian, *sukkal*) Isimud lets her in and tells Enki of her presence. The god greets her warmly, serves her butter cake, sweet water, and beer. Not just any beer, we recall, but "for my lady, emmer beer"—the most sacred beer. The two proceed to drink together; they "drink more and more beer" together. As Enki becomes drunkenly convivial, he begins to give the star goddess, one after another, the sets of laws that hold heaven and earth together. These laws are called the holy *me*.

With much toasting, Inanna accepts the laws, which are actually principles of civilization. More precisely, they are the gifts of royal menstrual office, beginning with the priestly offices, godship, kingship, and the high thrones, the underworld and its officers, and the sexual precincts, the crafts, and other elements of urban life. "I'll take it!" she exclaims after each offering. As eldest daughter of the moon couple, Inanna inherits the *me* by family right.

On and on the lists go, fourteen (lunar) sets of them, and the beer drinking goes on as well. Inanna accepts everything and loads the *me* into her Boat of Heaven. This boat appears in her love poetry as well, referring to her well-praised vulva; and of course it also refers to the world formation that derives from the vulva.

Leaving Enki in a drunken stupor, Inanna and her *sukkal,* Ninshubur, sail off in the direction of Inanna's city, Uruk. When Enki wakes up he calls out to Isimud in alarm. "Where is kingship?" he asks, "Where is decision?" "My lord," says the *sukkal,* "you have given them all to Inanna." Horrified as he realizes he has given away all the powers of rulership, Enki sends Isimud out over the water to get them back.

Inanna is enraged by what she calls Enki's deceit, and she calls on Ninshubur:

> Come, Ninshubur, once you were Queen of the East;
> Now you are the faithful servant of the holy shrine of Uruk.
> Water has not touched your hand,
> Water has not touched your foot.
> My *sukkal* who gives me wise advice,
> My warrior who fights by my side,
> Save the Boat of Heaven with the holy *me!* [10]

In the ensuing stormy water battles, Ninshubur, her hand slicing through the air, defeats a series of demons, monsters, and giants and even the "watchmen of the big canal" sent by Enki to sink the boat and recapture the *me*. On the day the Boat of Heaven arrives at Inanna's city, "High water swept over the streets/High water swept over the paths." But the high water is controlled, because the goddess has the menstrual laws in her possession.

The people of Uruk turn out for a festivity whose features are specified by the goddess: old men and old women are to give counsel and "heart-soothing"; young men must show their weapons; the high priest and the children will sing; and the king is to slaughter oxen and sheep and pour beer out of the cup; there is to be music of tambourines and people singing the praises of the goddess of the planet Venus.

Inanna sails her Boat of Heaven through the square gate of her city, flanked by her tall treelike emblems, and docks it in her own city's "white quay." Then she distributes the inherited *me* among all her people, adding a few more of her own: the spreading of the cloth on the ground, some feminine arts (of allure), and a new set of drums, including the kettledrum. And because this is a ritual passage of menstrual power, not a modern war with winners and losers, Enki then arrives at the celebration to bless his "daughter-in-law" Inanna and her city. She wins the right to the *me*, not because she is strongest and fiercest (though she is both), but because she is the most appropriate, as child of the moon she inherits the menstrual temple rites and, of course, the menstrual laws. The part Enki and his *sukkal* play is somewhat like that of the men in the mask lodges of tribal society, who dress as evil spirits to shake the menstrual hut, chase the initiated girls, and strike them, only to arrive much less fiercely marked at the great feast that announces the menstruants' emergence.

The high waters in this myth recede before the Boat of Heaven, and they are perhaps analogous to the carefully controlled waters of irrigation, at which Mesopotamian farmers excelled. The battle that rages between the powerful god of waters and a goddess of the sky is won by orientation itself. Venus is the Morning Star, and therefore Inanna is a point of orientation, especially of east. Nin-

217

shubur, as Queen of the East, is goddess of the dawn. She wins the battles with the chaotic forces for Inanna because she *is* East, the first knowable direction enacted millions of times at the emergence of menstruants from their seclusion into light.

As we saw earlier, in religious rites around the world, the four directions more than any other factor are what establish the idea "earth." Native American rites almost always include acknowledgment of the four earthly directions; this is done with body motions as well as in the construction of square altars. Less obviously but just as ritually, Jewish and Christian places of worship also make use of sacred direction and frequently emphasize east.

The Flood and Gilgamesh

A second Mesopotamian version of the menstrual flood and orientation myth shifts the central characters with their ark from two females to a man and his wife. From the area north of Sumer and south of the city of Babylon comes the Akkadian myth "The One Who Looked into the Abyss." The story is part of a long saga of King Gilgamesh, a historic figure whose reign is dated at around 2600 B.C.E. Fragments of this myth dating to a few centuries after the reign of the king exist, though the versions most repeated are from around 2000 B.C.E.[11]

King Gilgamesh and his companion Enkidu commit a grave transgression of protective taboo: they kill the guardian of the cedar forest in order to harvest the wood. (In addition, they mock Queen Ishtar, Inanna's Babylonian counterpart). A committee of deities decide to kill Enkidu, but they spare Gilgamesh. The king is so distraught by his friend's death that he cannot participate in the normal mourning rites and instead embarks on a journey to learn the nature of death and immortality. Along his way, Gilgamesh reaches the shore of the sea of death, the dwelling of a female guardian (or priestess) whose title is the "Bar Maid" (or Alewife). Gilgamesh tells the Bar Maid his fear that death is a finality. She, true to the courtesan (and barmaid) tradition, listens to his question and then instructs him how to cross the sea between life and death. She sends him to the boatman, who says that he can take him across the sea in a journey of three days, providing he does not "touch the waters with his hand." At his next landing, Gilgamesh stays with a figure named Utnapishtim, who tells him the Flood story.

This portion of the Gilgamesh epic created a sensation when it was first translated in the nineteenth century, for until then few in the Christian West recognized that many biblical stories derive from myths thousands of years older than those collected as the Old Testament. In this earliest known written version, some elemental gods gather to discuss the possibility of sending humankind a flood, not as a punishment, simply as an event. The first deities listed are Mama, the great water (Tiamat), and An, the sky, then the storm god Enlil, followed by a throne-bearer and an inspector of irrigation canals. Ishtar/Inanna is also present, as is last-named Ea, the Word who is able to enter the underworld. Since Ea is also Enki, two of the deities in the Sumerian Boat of Heaven myth are present in the Babylonian Flood story as well. These deities all have a direct association with the fundamental elements of menstrual creation, including the "throne-bearer," who can control the cosmic waters by enabling the gods to sit safely off the earth, and the inspector of irrigation canals, whose engineering tasks would have also been religious concerns in the equation of the canal and the vagina.

But without agreement of the council of deities, the storm god Enlil capriciously proceeds to rain a deluge. Before the rains begin, Ea learns of the impending disaster. He goes first to the *giparu*, the holy reed hut, and addresses the walls of it to warn the human Utnapishtim, instructing him what to do when the rain begins: "Tear down the house. Build an ark./Abandon riches, seek life!" says Ea, telling him to load the seed of every living thing into it.[12]

The descriptions of the ark fit a building rather than a water-

219

going vessel. The sides are high, there are three stories, no keel, no prow. Perhaps it is called a boat because it derives from Inanna's Boat of Heaven, the arc of the crescent moon. The ark in the Gilgamesh epic is no longer a "vulva boat," but its detailed measurements suggest its metaformic dimension. It is perfectly square, ten dozen cubits on each side. The ark is thus a geometrical shape. Inanna had the Queen of the East and the vulva; perhaps the male survivor of the Flood must have another method of measurement, a metaform that will let him form solid ground and make his way about on it. Perhaps that metaform is a structure holding the idea of squareness, the four directions in complete alignment. Moreover, the ark covers "an acre" of floorspace, so it is a unit of farmland in area. The sacred number of menstrual creation is connected to both the ark and the flood: the ark is in seven levels (with nine inner parts); it takes seven days to build; there are seven days of storm, and it takes seven days for the ark to land on the mountaintop. Three birds are sent out to search for land, and the four winds are sent out as well.

Ea's warning, "Say that at dawn he will rain down bread, he will rain wheat," can be read ironically. But we also know the equation of wheat with rain has deeper significance, for wheat—especially red, emmer wheat, from which sacred beer was made—is a powerful metaform. Utnapishtim lists how lavishly he feeds his workmen. In addition to butchering bulls and sheep, every day they swill beer, wine, and oil—as though for the New Year feast day, he says. Again our attention is caught by menstrual associations.

The committee of gods are horrified at the destruction of humanity on earth, and they blame Enlil for taking matters into his own hands without finalizing the plan with the rest of them. In their distress, they establish a new law of justice based in individual responsibility: let only the one who is guilty be punished, and not the whole human race, or any group. Ea speaks the covenant: henceforth death shall not come in the form of Flood. Death will be more selective in keeping human population within bounds, and

220

to that end Ea decrees only four ills to diminish humankind: the lion, the wolf, famine, and the plague.

The Ark and the Covenant of Yahweh

The Flood myth in Genesis was written down about two thousand years after King Gilgamesh reigned in Erech, and after his story had been copied so many times that it may have been the most popular of the Mesopotamian myths. The Genesis version of the Flood establishes one of the most crucial covenants of the Hebrew religion, and of Christianity as well. Islam also has a version in the Koran, though much sparser in detail than the earlier myths.

In Genesis, Utnapishtim and his wife have become Noah and his wife, the only female element remaining. Ea, Mama, Enlil, Ishtar, and the whole committee of Babylonian creation goddess and gods are now merged into one, Yahweh, who sends the rain not on a whim of rage, but deliberately to destroy humankind because it has become "violent and corrupt." The ark again has carefully delineated dimensions, and again, it is clearly not a boat.[13]

The covenant between Yahweh and Noah, and all his seed and "every living creature that is of flesh," is the Rainbow:

> And I will establish my covenant with you; neither shall all flesh be cut off any more by the waters of a flood; neither shall there any more be a flood to destroy the earth. And God said, This is the token of the covenant which I make between me and you and every living creature that is with you, for perpetual generations: I do set my bow in the cloud, and it shall be for a token of a covenant between me and the earth.[14]

Humanity's part of the covenant is to remember the successful landing of the ark of Noah when Yahweh sets the Rainbow arc in the sky.

In Exodus there is a detailed description of yet another ark, the ark of the covenant, and of the tabernacle that encloses it. Both

221

Flood Stories and Menstrual Rite: Common Elements

	Orientation	Ark	Chair	Food
Menstrual Seclusion	East, light	Womb, vulva, hut	Log, stool	Water, grain
Inanna/Enki	Queen of East	Boat of Heaven	High throne	Red beer, cake
Utnapishtim/Ea	Mountaintop	*Giparu* & square ark	Throne-bearer	Beer, bread
Noah/Yahweh	Mountain	Rectangular ark	(Yahweh's throne)	* *
Ark of the Covenant	East side veiled	Rectangular box & Tabernacle	Seat of mercy	Showbread

became incorporated into the Jewish temple. The ark is an oblong box made of acacia wood enclosed in gold, resting within a wooden three-sided structure that is veiled on its east side with lushly colored linen cloth. This tabernacle is itself enclosed within a cloth tent. Thus both the metaformic square of orientation and the first direction are retained in a place of seclusion. According to Exodus, inside the ark are the Lord's testimony, tables of laws, the rod of Aaron, and a pot of manna. On top of the ark rests, according to careful specifications, the "seat of mercy," over which stand two cherubim with their wings protectively covering the chair, which is in "the most holy place." [15] Inside the tabernacle is a table on which is the showbread; the priest alone may enter the Holy of Holies where the ark is kept, and then only after a blood sacrifice.

Using the menstrual elements of chair, birds, flood, blood, and the four directions, the ancient Hebrews put narrative itself into the wooden ark, orienting their lives around written law and written myth. To a great extent, story alone would guide their travels on the face of the hard, still earth, with the help of the tabernacle's veiled face, always aimed toward the east.

Covenant	Contents	Birds	Serpent
World-formation, no flood	Taboos	Two doves taken for sacrifice	Snake & rainbow
Blessing & peace after storm	Fourteen sets of *me*	Flying giants	(Inanna's snake)
No flood	Seeds & animals, silver & gold	Dove, swallow, crow	(Inanna's snake)
No flood	Seeds & animals	Dove, raven	Rainbow
No flood	Torah	Two winged cherubim	Multi-colored cloth

Words with roots related to tabernacle include "table," not only the square or rectangular shape considered a prerequisite for formal dining and alter alike, but also tables of numbers, the writing tablet, and—shades of the Alewife—the word "tavern." The mountain that Noah's ark landed upon is Mount Ararat, the more northerly spelling of which is Ararath, or Earth. Hera's name may be read there, and Sara's, bringing the mythic female back into the story.[16]

In the biblical Flood myth, it was a white dove that ultimately found dry land. White doves, as I have said, are metaforms for the new moon, and in the Near East the white dove had explicit connections to menstrual rite. The text of Leviticus, which spells out the seven-day menstrual seclusion, also requires that on the eighth day after her seclusion a woman must take two turtledoves or young pigeons to the priest for sacrificial atonement for her uncleanness.[17] Again and again, the practices of menstrual seclusion surface in the ancient myths of humankind. My chart of the Flood myths (above) displays their overlapping elements and the recurrent metaforms of menstrual rite.

223

The Flood myth is the covenant between humans and universal mind, the promise that through external measurement—for some peoples the Rainbow Snake and for others the orientation of the *giparu,* the sacred hut-womb and ark—we will not be lost. We will not be helpless victims of watery chaos. The Flood myth promised that the "menstruation" of the sky—whether the monsoon (moon's rain) or the seasonal overflowing of rivers and lakes—would not overwhelm our ancestors, who had come to understand that dry land would inevitably appear again. Their recognition of cycles, of orientation—the ark that bears direction, sacred number, astronomical observation, and the seeds and *me* of civilization—assured us that we could always begin again, no mater how far we fled in terror or what landmarks had been washed away. In this view, the Flood myth says that external measurement is our connection to deity, and it also is the basis of our science. The promise that we could rely on human mind, could leave so much instinct behind and not perish in chaos, has never been broken.

These narrative metaforms, products of the evolving menstrual *logos,* gradually replaced physical ritual, so that origin story itself "crossed over" from the female to the male principle. It has been said that the menstrual tradition is "a river of blood" connecting all women. Heros often have to cross mythic rivers to attain their goals, and in narrative, too, men had to cross the Abyss in order to identify with what had formerly been entirely female protagonists.

Using "and," the simplest metaphoric connection, people constructed compound oral narratives, describing their rites and incorporating sacred number, orientation, and wilderness and food metaforms. They used as plots the menstrual *logos,* the journeys that retold the course of the menstruant. Raised to her greatest logic of inclusion, she encompassed the constellations and the sun, moon, and earth. From her characterizations as primal creator, we understood deity as having a human visage, human emotions, and human motives while remaining connected to more ancient wilderness metaforms. Her combined forms, often imagined as male-female or sister-brother pairs, filled the great pantheons of ancient

224

religions, from Greece and Mesopotamia to West and North Africa, China, Japan, Southeast Asia, the South Pacific, northern Europe, North America among the Pueblos, and further south with the Inca and the Maya. In their writing down, the narratives of creation would gradually cross the genders, changing from all-female to all-male stories over a period of about two thousand years. Increasingly, narrative metaforms replaced *cosmetikos* as the central Word communicating origins.

If the earliest "writings" were sacred numbers and chevrons carved or tatooed into the menstruant's flesh, these markings then migrated onto her clothing and the surfaces of woman-shaped pots, and finally, as an alphabet, the marks migrated to clay tablets. We could say that Word migrated from skin to skirt, from skirt to script. The Sumerians were not the only people to develop writing, of course. Chinese writing evolved from divinatory markings on bones, and it continues to modernize as the world changes. Ancient Egyptian hieroglyphs and Mayan temple writings continue to puzzle researchers and to reveal the past. But the abstraction of alphabet systems of the ancient Middle East spread writing across languages and cultures, unifying people of very diverse backgrounds and geographical areas, and enabling a new kind of logic—written discourse. For five thousand years, written metaform has spread across the world, retaining and conveying humanity's knowledge.

In conjunction with the spread of written creation stories, another kind of metaform, *material metaform,* also began to take center stage. How it gave us the underpinnings of our modern lives, why male-only origin stories have been so dominant, and where we might be going next are questions I address in the next section: Roses.

Part Four

. . . R O S E S . . .
Material Metaform

■ ■ ■ ■ ■ ■ ■ ■ ■ ■ ■

Chapter 14

Crafting the Earth's Menstruation: Materialism

T H E Babylonian myth of King Gilgamesh and his complex struggles with Queen Ishtar, her underworld, and the epic flood, opens with a special creation story. The goddess Aruru makes a man by pinching a bit of red clay. This act of creation is not one of thought, or of separation, rather it is an act of creation through handcraft, manufacture. The myth anticipates a new era of social organization: the city, whose foundations are in the menstrual economies of farming, herding, and horticulture, but whose ritual emphasis is on the making of crafts—not only pottery, but metallurgy, jewelry, carving, carpentry, and the multitude of material manipulations that have become engineering. The crafts are given a full listing in the *me* that Inanna receives into her Boat of Heaven: the woodworker, copper worker, scribe, smith, leather worker, fuller, builder, and reed worker. Craftsmen were so completely integrated into the goddess religion that in India, "five classes of artisans—the carpenters, the gold smiths, the blacksmiths, the brass-smiths, and masons—regarded themselves as the original creators of form and called themselves *Brahmin kammalars*. They insisted on their right to enact the sacred rituals. In village societies, the craftsman was the officiating magician-priest at the shrine of the goddess."[1]

Regardless of how lost my Swedish-born father seems to get in modern America, he is always centered in his skill and love of wood carving. His craft always brings him back together within himself after another failure of lady luck has shattered him. Whenever he is fired or laid off work, he sits home drinking pots of coffee, humming and carving. He shapes miniature figures and sailing ships, little brass cannon, slender six-inch-long scale models of Civil War rifles. He also reads history books and tells me stories about Europe and other places—with special attention to the trees and kinds of wood in each location—so his carvings seem a sort of profound meditation on his own origins.

I don't have the knack of carving, though at twelve I try; the first thing I carve is, oddly enough, a little coiled snake. I give it a hat and bow tie to hide my embarrassment at its simplicity with a bit of humor. But my father still has given me craft: the understanding that creativity comes from concentration and inner stillness—a kind of listening to and honoring the sources and materials of one's own artful discipline. Very simple tools are all that is needed. He uses a razor-sharp pocket knife, a pencil, scraps of wood, metal, or plastic, found in trash heaps, and tiny bottles of paint. His tool chest is a cardboard box kept under his side of the little bed he shares with my mother. Because of him, I have a deep respect for the making of objects.

If the ancestral protohumans were strange animals who spent millennia learning to wear matted skirts and long hats, how much stranger still that their descendants sat hunched for millions of hours over bits of cord, wood, metal, and clay, forming them into shapes imitative of those they saw in life. Why, they might have wondered, do we do this? To investigate the relationship of crafts and menstruation, I begin by considering one of the oddest of them: the rose. Although it lives, the rose, like a multitude of handmade objects, is a product of human skill. It has been crafted through horticulture. That people would take so much time and trouble to cultivate such a prickly, uncomfortable, inedible plant, dragging it with them to every new place of living, across sea and land, building hothouses and raised beds simply in order to gaze upon its blooms seems odd behavior indeed.

The rose is a venerable symbol of love and, more fundamentally, of the vulva, blood red. Roses are given on occasions to express love and respect. Thousands of people spend their lives breeding, raising, arranging, and selling roses. The trade in roses and other flowers is itself a small economy as there are over ten thousand varieties of roses. The rose, originating in Persia, stemmed from Arab cultures and spread throughout Christianized Europe. It became a primary symbol of Mary, who is often called "the Rose," "Rose-garden," "Mystic Rose," and the like. Gothic cathedrals featured a rose window, situated in the west, a counterpoint to the male cross in the eastern apse.[2]

Given that a Neanderthal grave contained pollen, suggesting that flowers were sprinkled there, the question arises of why human attention should have turned to such an odd thing as a flower? Flowers are mythically significant worldwide, the tropical reds of Hawaiian flowers, the lotus of India. It is hard to imagine the poems of classical Japan without the image of flowering plum. And for other peoples, the poppy, carnation, tulip, chrysanthemum, poinsettia, and other flowers selected for brilliant red coloring are objects of great attention. Elaborate festivals from India to Southeast Asia are resplendent with flower offerings, and religious altars around the world overflow with flowers.

The rose is thus only one of many metaformic flowers, but it is one of the most powerful. I call the rose a "craft," because though it is something cultivated and harvested, it isn't a food or herb. Its value lies in the significance of its form, in what we call its beauty, its *cosmetikos*. The smell, color, shape, number of petals and thorns of the rose all contribute to a metaformic statement of the bleeding vulva—of the plant world.

The gnostic Gospels, dated around four hundred years after Christ, contain an origin story of the rose and of flowers in general that is overtly menstrual. In the context of romantic love, the

231

story associates the menstruation of humans and "menstruations" of plant life:

> But the first Psyche (Soul) loved Eros who was with her, and poured her blood upon him and upon the earth. Then from that blood the rose first sprouted upon the earth out of the thorn bush, for a joy in the light which was to appear in the bramble. After this the beautiful, fragrant flowers sprouted up in the earth according to their kind from the blood of each of the virgins of the daughters of Pronoia. When they had become enamored of Eros, they poured out their blood upon him and upon the earth. After these things, every herb sprouted up in the earth according to kind.[3]

Pronoia is a female substance, translated as "foreknowledge." From the menstrual blood of the daughters of foreknowledge came the rose as token of their love for Eros, god of sexual love. And from the exuberance of their expression came plant life on earth— which I take to mean human use of, or cultivation of, garden plants.

In Leviticus, the biblical chapter of regulatory laws governing behavior, a woman's period is called her "flowers". "And if her flowers be upon her . . ." or "And of her that is sick of her flowers . . ."[4] On this continent, too, menstruation was called "flowers." A Yurok myth says that Coyote created menstruation and menstrual laws, and the human culture hero helped this process by cutting his ankle and smearing blood on a girl's thigh, whereupon Coyote said, "You got flowers now."[5] Barbara Walker has pointed out that the word flower is literally "flow-er," menstruator, and in much of the European tradition as well, menstruation was once called "flowers." Old English forms related to *blod*, "blood," are *blowan, blew,* and *blown,* meaning "to bloom, to blossom." In French, *fluer* means "flow," and *fleurs,* "flowers." And in German the singular *Blut* is blood while the plural *Blüte* is flower; in Hungarian *vér* is blood, *veres* is red, and *vér-ag* is bloom, flower. The Karok of California held a special "flower dance" in summer for girls who had begun to menstruate. An approving Spanish name for lesbians is *las flores,* "the flowers," used among some families of North America. Women are often named for flowers, and many goddesses have special flowers. The rose was the flower of Sappho's goddess, Aphrodite, a latter-day Inanna. And Inanna's eight-pointed symbol is called a rosette and was sometimes depicted growing on a tree or vine.[6]

The smell of roses is one method of cleaning the taint of shame, associated with the smell of menstrual blood, which has attached itself to the female body. When the rose is worn as a perfume it is *cosmetikos*, part of female allure that says, "See how well I take care of myself, for your benefit." When the rose is used as a cut flower, carried or worn, it is more of a craft, a metaform replacing and purifying the vulva's image. The bride's entire body is veiled in cloth, her sexuality not even suggested by her garb; yet she may carry the round red bridal bouquet, the collective floral vulva, to pass on to the next most marriageable maiden. No blood needs to show at the modern wedding or festival, but red flowers are a common substitute, their petals torn and scattered over the table, the punch bowl, the carpet, and the bridal chair, like the blood drops scattered on the queenly throne in Inanna's New Year's procession.

The rose was metaformically crafted from menstrual blood and is associated with controlled sexual love. The presentation of a rose is a form of speech, a word passing between any two people who desire connection, but particularly between a man and woman. Traditionally, when men bring roses to women, women feel cherished. The flowers release feelings of tenderness and romance. People also use the scent of flowers to equalize our smells—perhaps a political necessity as local village populations became mass urban populations, enormous groups of strangers. The rose and similar flowers became prized trade objects. One early capitalist enterprise, in Holland, consisted of speculations in the sale of tulip bulbs. But long before the Dutch discovered the profits of flowers; perfumed oils and rose waters were products of frequent exchange in the shipping trades of Egypt and Phoenicia, Persia and Greece.

The rose is also a *token* of love, a "payment" to the menstrual/ erotic mind itself and traded between hearts. How did this come

233

about, that we would use flowers as a kind of payment? And just what do we mean by "payment"?

Trade, Payment, and the Ant Mound

I discussed earlier how the Dogon's threshing of the *fonio* grain at night is a way of paying the earth her due for the knowledge of incest and in atonement for (recognition of) the jackal's negative character. Other ideas of payment, trade, and the exchange of crafts are also connected to the menstrual mind at the heart of human culture. The Dogon origin story of trade begins with twins. The very first trade, Ogotemmêli says, began when twins sat down on the red ant mound. The two sat down on the mound of the earth's menstruating vulva and exchanged two kinds of words: cloth and cowrie shells, each of which is a metaform for living language. Twinness is a cornerstone of Dogon philosophy for many reasons, but one is that twins gave the Dogon people the underlying idea of trade, the idea of the essential equality of two unique objects. In trade, the cloth and the cowries are equalized; that is to say, negotiations continue until the two elements are "twinned." Twinness teaches, at the same time it embodies, the mathematical idea of equation. For the Dogon, this idea exists in the context of menstrual balance of powers: the life/death character of the red ant mound.[7]

Cloth, as decorated skin, had unimaginable value to people for whom it was a metaform. In Africa, cloth making reached heights of color and design, especially geometric design, and had ritual significance equaled only in a few other places—among the indigenous people of Central America and in parts of Asia, for example. Cowrie shells are used for divination in religious rites as well as in trade. Rounded like a pregnant belly on one side and with a deep vulva on the other, the delicate shells are obvious female metaforms, though some peoples consider them male on one side and female on the other. The cowries are a means of divining information from the gods, of calling them through their sacred numbers,

234

by casting that precise number of shells. The means of barter is also a means of prayer or instruction between human and universal mind, for the cowries are considered words and accompany verbal communication.

In Dogon society, and throughout most of the traditional village world, the most important element of trade is the verbal exchange that precedes the transaction and that establishes price. The Dogon consider that the cloth and the cowries both have spirit and are both alive; they speak to each other through the mouths of the human traders. According to Ogotemmêli, cloth itself is full of words—from the art of spinning (which comes from the mouths of women) and of weaving (which the men now do, and which has ancestral narrative significance). There are also words in the designs, deriving as they do from *cosmetikos*. The cowries of payment are thus a form of language, as is the cloth. Trade, then, may be thought of as speaking, a form of communication that spreads the "goods" of words among the population.

Payment for an object owned by someone else *cleans* it. The Dogon believe that a spirit of the owner attaches to his or her property, so if you borrow something, the owner's essence clings to it and causes future trouble. All tribal peoples understand this, and so do psychics in the West. Trade, or paying fair price for the object, first equalizes the exchange, then wipes out this clinging spirit essence so there is no "debt," no interfering presence of the original owner. The object is washed clean by the exchange of value for value, ready to be enfused with the spirit of the new owner. Payment may be understood as a method of balancing menstrual powers by "cleaning" out old influences, re-newing. The original twins of trade sat on the red ant mound and learned the menstrual arts of measuring, speaking, equalizing, and renewing—establishing a "flow" of trade.

These associations are acknowledged even now in industrial society. When negotiations go wrong, people describe the feeling as "dirty": the deal "smells bad," we got a "raw deal," or there is something "fishy," that is, menstrual, about it. We feel proud when we can pay for something with our "own" money or when we are "free and clear" of debt. Appropriately paid for objects are "goods." Goods not paid for are stolen, dirtied. They must be paid for in more drastic ways, perhaps in blood, perhaps by restriction—years of forced separation from others, in some societies in small cages where the prisoner is fed "bread and water," the menstrual seclusion food of simple jail fare.

On the tribal California coast, shells, often round white ones, were used as money. They can clearly be related to the full, or nonmenstruating, moon. But given that the Kogi people associate white shells with the semen of their male creation sky god, there may also have been a male principle underlying the use of white shells on the northern continent. Red woodpecker scalps were another form of money among California tribes, and some young men collected long strings of the little scarlet patches. Early in this century, a Yurok woman named Weitchpec Susie reported that postmenstrual "washing" in the center of the sky, the cleanest possible place, attained by following "paths" made of woodpecker heads, dentalia shells, and white deerskin (all highly valued), would make a woman rich all her life.[8]

The word "money" comes from moon—"mooney"—and in ancient Rome the mint was in the temple of Juno, goddess of marriage. In all likelihood round coins made of silver and other metals were sometimes portraits of the full moon and sun. Gold and silver coins were equated with semen in some European folk songs. Coins are still used as *cosmetikos* by many peoples. They form women's marriage headdresses throughout the Middle East and adorn special skirts of sexual allure worn by women dancers, and in the West, money is still tucked into the G-strings of sexual dancers.

In the Mesopotamian region, even as city-states developed, the priestess class continued the sacred ideas underlying trade. The roots of a money economy were established within the temples themselves, for trade had religious significance. The supplicant brought a lunar/seminal payment—metaforms such as shells, salt, coins, precious gems, or metals—in exchange for a blessing of some sort, whether a prayer, a rite, a sexual exchange, the sacrifice of a cow.

The rose, like other selected crafts, is a substitution for blood payment, the blood that poured from Psyche, the first embodiment of foreknowledge. Blood drops were metaformically transformed into rose petals. I think of payment as a debt of recognition; we are kept conscious of our origins by the act of paying. Payment also exchanges the former owner's essence for one's own by equalizing and washing the object. This trading, or "speaking" through trading, has largely replaced blood sacrifice (although we see how quickly in mass society, groups left out of the process of trade resort to bloodshed to make themselves heard). The roots of modern materialist society thus lie in the metaforms through which people began to "speak" by trading significant crafts.

Mineral Metaforms

Australian myths still recall the origin of red ochre deposits as the spilling of menstrual blood by ancestral dancers, and it is a logical extension that ancient peoples would have used the menstrual mind to order the strata of the earth's mineral composition. Not only streams of water, springs, rivers, and the sea were first comprehended through images of blood (and analogous body fluids), but also the minerals of the earth.

Metals and gems of ancient smiths and jewelers had religious significance connected to women's blood and the earth's blood, even the "blood" of the sun. The Dogon consider the red metal copper to be an excretion of the sun, which is female. They also associate copper with water, perhaps because of the green appearance of the "raw" ore. All manner of taboos surround the art of smithing in their villages. For example, because the smith stole fire from the sun, his fire is a piece of sun, and he must not do his work after sunset.[9] Copper is metaphorically associated with fluid, and even late in the Western tradition, less than two hundred years ago, fire, too, was considered to be a fluid. Iron ore—red and smelling

237

like blood, which also has iron content, is ringed with taboos. Among some peoples, it cannot touch the earth, for instance. For others, it fashions the protective stool or shoes that are placed between a royal menstruant and the vulnerable earth.

The primary stones used in the *cosmetikos* of the temple priestesses and the goddess Inanna/Ishtar of Mesopotamia were lapis lazuli and carnelian, both considered blood of the earth. As a red stone, carnelian is more obvious, but deep blue lapis, too, was menstrual and is named in the Bible as *sappur*, "holy blood." [10] In the narrative of Inanna's descent to underworld seclusion, her body is compared to three materials of the craftsman: boxwood, a wood used to make ornaments to cover the vulva; silver, an exudate of the moon; and lapis lazuli, the earth's menstruation. [11] The Kogi people of Colombia describe all veins of minerals as the Mother's blood, as they do underground water. The fact that blue and green stones were considered "blood" makes more sense if we remember that the metaphoric mind was relating them to the life-giving waters of the earth, and treating watery images as blood was a method of organizing complex ideas. Jade, too, the "heavenly stone" of China, which in its "raw" form is crusted with red, can be associated with blood. The Kogi believe that gold itself is menstrual blood, that mining is the same as draining the Mother's life-giving streams, and that the whole ecosystem of plant and cloud life is threatened by the materialist exploitation of the earth. [12]

If gold and other minerals are the blood of the earth, clay is her flesh. Kogi taboos regarding clayworkers are clues as to how they, and other ancient farming cultures, must have used menstrual seclusion laws to learn to work gold, silver, and other minerals. While women may have first created pottery, among the Kogi it is the men who do it. They believe that "an earthenware jar is one more aspect of the womb-mother." [13] The care with which they approach the craft of pottery as a menstrual rite reflects also how their forefathers approached gold smithing (which is no longer done). "Women do not need a great effort of spiritual preparation to make a *mochila* [woven bag] because every woman is in a sense the Mother. But pots are made by men. Men must approach the making of a pot with as much care and seriousness as they approach the coming of manhood." [14] The potter digs clay for four days (the sacred number); he eats no salt; he cannot look at women or enter the house of a woman; he bathes only at night. He keeps strictly to these regulations the entire time in which he makes pots, a designated period of one month. And in keeping with the menstrual tradition, a trade payment is necessary: "The clay of the earth was a woman. That is why when a Mama is going to have a pot made he has to make a payment" of a small white stone. [15]

The Kogi and other precolombian peoples made figurines of gold, sometimes keeping them in their fields. Small gold or clay statues of goddess figures were a common feature in old agricultural cultures—in the valley of Mexico as well as the Near East, in Crete, Malta, Eastern Europe, as well as in prechristian Greece, and many other places. One purpose of such figurines is made clear by contemporary rural villagers in India, who say that the little clay statues in their fields are substitutes for human sacrifice, part of an old earth religion. Not so long ago, they would have killed members of their own families and put their dismembered bodies in the fields to guarantee the crop. [16]

For ancient craftworkers, gold had a sacred value, not a commercial worth. The gold figurines that Kogi ancestors placed in graves, fields, and temples usually represented the earth Mother—though there were Snake forms also—and the little padded female figures wear big earrings, like an emergent menstruant. The figurines were always stored in clay pots, which was entirely logical, since gold was equated with menstrual blood and clay pots with wombs. The Kogi also kept precious gems and gold in stone temples for protection—just as the royal menstruants were kept behind thick stone walls in kingdoms all around the Northern Hemisphere and in Mayan cities, in Egypt, and in all probability in other African kingdoms as well.

Since craftspeople considered gems, silver, and gold to be the Mother's menstrual blood and clay to be her flesh, the "purification" of any of these substances with fire was menstrual logic, an extension of their religious structure, leading directly to the crafts of metallurgy, smithing, and fired pottery. Throughout the Middle Ages, alchemists chased the possibility of transmuting all manner of minerals into gold, and in the course of this essentially menstrual exercise, at which they systematically failed, they discovered the basics of what has become modern chemistry.

Engineering also developed, as the tools and ideas used in *cosmetikos* were transferred to crafts. Indeed, we might think of crafts as the *cosmetikos* of the earth: trees are carved as skin was carved; clay is "the same as" flesh; pins hold flesh, pins hold cloth, pins hold clay. Crafts were in this way an expansion of human mind outside the body.

When the decorations of *cosmetikos* migrated off the body, they would as a matter of course have been translated into the forms and functions used in mechanics—most obviously, as we have seen, in cords and strings, from umbilical cords and cat's cradle. Objects designed to be embedded in ear lobes and lips were geometric and shaped with grooved edges and interlocking parts. From *cosmetikos*, the essential shapes and functions for external equipment—the grooved disk, the double-headed knob, the belt, the trapezoid, globe, and triangle shapes—developed. These were all forms that some societies would come to use in mechanical devices, as linch and cotter pins, pegs, wedges, dowels, swivels, and nails. Both genders participated in the formation of engineering, as the shapes had passed over to the men through their puberty and marriage ceremonies, for men, too, used lip plugs and ear plugs and other elaborate embedded body adornment, including smooth wooden pins inserted in the penis. The fundamental shapes of *cosmetikos* are seen in the mechanics of block and tackle, pulley, spool, gear, winch, and wheel that turned waterwheels, lifted stones, hoisted sails, and built temples and houses.

The paraphernalia of the menstrual hut, too, contained the elements of engineering and design: the scratching stick that separated the menstruant's contaminated fingers from the earth of her skin would scratch the surface of the earth itself as digging stick or hoe. In male hands, it would later become a plow, identified in myth with the penis: "Plow my vulva, man of my heart!"[17] The mortar and pestle is the structure of the ball and socket that swung doors of cities in Sumer. The mats that seated the menstruant off the earth became the molds for clay plates and other utensils. The swan- or eagle-bone straw became, among other things, the flute, played by young men in many cultures to woo women. The greatly cherished cow or bull horn of the African or Teutonic chief—blown at the New Moon, kept in a cloistered place and polished with sacred oil—can be heard today as the trumpets with which men continue to speak to the Mystery.

Taberna: The Sacred Tavern

My parents greatest point of disparity was over my father's love of drinking, not only his inability to stop and his atrocious, boring behavior when drunk, but also that it kept him away from home. My father loved the tavern and the company of other men, the convivial conversations, the music and gambling, and the big-handed gestures of buying "drinks on the house." He probably liked the convivial women there as well, but that was never discussed in front of me. I grew up ambivalent toward drinking, periodically imitating my father in doing it and my mother in stopping it. Some ancient people treated drunkenness as an illness, and common menstrual law would have prohibited pregnant and nursing women from imbibing. The Dogon completely prohibit adults from drinking until they are old, and then it is expected of them, and people listen closely to drunken elders as the voices of spirits in prophecy. I like this system best, and look forward to being a raving lush in my seventies and eighties.

The words "tavern" and "tabernacle" both derive from Latin *taberna*, hut. The diminutive is "tent" and the first *Websters Dictionary* definition of tabernacle is "a tent sanctuary used by the Isra-

241

elites during the Exodus." Tabernacle also means a "receptacle for the consecrated elements of the Eucharist," especially an "ornamental locked box fixed to the middle of the altar and used for reserving the host." Finally, tabernacles are houses of worship, such as a tent or large building for evangelistic services. The secular place of gathering and drinking alcohol is "tavern," and in modern Greek the earlier pronunciation "taberna" refers to a cafe.

A tavern today is a public place to go to enjoy oneself, to drink with others and achieve an altered state of mind and spirit, perhaps to meet a sexual partner or to pour out one's troubles to the sympathetic bartender. In ancient Sumerian practice, the elements were the same; but they were treated as sacred *r'tu*. A special bed for the harlot goddess Inanna was made in the tavern, making it a place of sacred "one-night matrimony." From as early as 4000 B.C.E., Sumerian men were depicted dressed in floor-length skirts and carefully seated "off the earth" on chairs, sharing big jars of beer, which they drank through long straws, perhaps made of lapis lazuli and gold. Such straws were found at Ur in the grave of Lady Pu-abi dated at around 2600 B.C.E. Alewives owned the taverns, trading beer for silver coins. (The code of Hammurabi specified they were to be drowned for overcharging.)

The tavern premises were tabooed to high priestesses, who as the ultimate menstrual figure would have interfered with its powers—setting off natural disasters, of which flood was the most likely and logical. A hymn to Ninkasi, the beer goddess, makes clear that sacred flowing waters and sacred beer are metaformically related. Ninkasi's mother is called "the sacred lake," the fermenting yeast is likened to the sea ("the waves rise/the waves fall"), and the final pouring of the filtered red liquid is equated to the onrushing waters of the Tigris and Euphrates Rivers, those two sisterly flows.[18]

The Sumerian *taberna* was a place of "crossing over," as alewives offered the foaming metaform to the public, that is to say, to men. It is easy to see how the tabernacle came to be a box or other container holding consecrated bread and wine of sacred rite. The tavern is a secular version of some of the oldest sacraments, and in all probability the drinking men practiced divination and prophetic speech as part of their rite. Skoal, Dad.

From Taberna to Temple

Like the tavern and the tabernacle, the temple evolved from the basic hut of menstrual orientation into a structure where more complex measurements of time and space were kept. The word "temple" has roots in "time"—as do "tempo," "temporary," and "contemplation"—from Latin *tempus,* "time," and *templum,* "space marked out for the observation of auguries." It is also related to *tempestas,* "season" or "storm." What besides time has been kept in temples? Orientation, statuary, ritual paraphernalia, fire, water, books, grain, fruits, cattle, money, and crafts. As temples became centers of trade, the earliest known cities grew up around them.

It is entirely likely that the menstrual hut, as the original dwelling, was the axis around which the village grew. The menstrual hut was not only oriented toward light, but also direction and major landscape features, such as rivers, lakes, and springs. A map of typical North American Indian hunting and gathering villages shows that menstrual huts were placed *near* a river or stream, but *away* from the spring or source of drinking water, thus marking the difference between drinking water and washing water.[19] The Dogon village is laid out in an oval and imagined as a human body; two women's houses, the menstrual huts, are just outside the oval and on its east-west axis; they are round and are called the "hands" of the village. In the north, inside the oval, is a square shelter for the men. These two structures are the first ones built in a new village.[20] Conversely, menstrual huts may be the last structure abandoned in a village. In one African tribe, the menstrual hut was located in an older village, and women journeyed from the new village to the older, keeping its history.

Menstrual practices established areas as sacred: In Hawaii,

women used old skirts as menstrual pads, which they sometimes stuffed into the cracks of the slatted house, or *hale*. Men refused to lean against the side of a house lest they accidentally touch one of the used pads. More often, women buried their pads in areas around the seclusion huts, and these areas were taboo, forming sacred precincts into which no one except menstruating women would go.[21] Sacred ground surrounds most temples, and it is possible that the habit of setting apart all the ground around seclusion huts can account for it. Among many peoples, both menstruation and birthing huts were burned or abandoned after a single use, and the area was then taboo. This must have given women phenomenal practice at house building, as well as establishing specific "off limits" territory, "sacred ground" associated with the primal house of orientation and origin.

Most ancient Greek temples used the central idea of the grove of trees holding up the sky. By substituting stone for wood, the Greeks devised the polished and painted marble column to hold up the roofs of their temples. Even with so much marble, the rituals practiced within the temples were not far from the menstrual hut of reeds and grass. On annual feasting occasions, reclining couches were replaced with crude beds of twigs, and small temple houses were replaced with specially built rude huts, as though participants were enacting *the way back* to earlier forms of the temple.[22] The feast of Hera, featured structures of pine or willow branches, the feast of Olympia, olive branches.[23]

The earliest Greek temple, according to Carl Kerényi, was that of Hera, and it was a prototype for the later, more "Olympian" structures. Hera's temple at Samos does not at all resemble a hut. As I said earlier, it is more a long vaginal cave or underworld, or an enclosed path through the woods—a long, narrow, dark chamber, with a line of columnar "trees" down the center. The goddess in her shape as a slab of oak, stayed in seclusion at the dark end of her stone temple, as if in a forested underworld.

Because the royal menstruant represented the collective metaformic mind, royal burials were associated with the essential "hut" of orientation—the temple, the palace, and the sacred precincts around them. The lunar, solar, and stellar alignments of temples worldwide is well documented, not only of monumental stone edifices but of simple sacred constructions: some peoples used simple poles pointed to the North Pole, or made a line drawing to mark the falling of sun rays into the back of a cave at the summer or winter solstice.

The underlying menstrual imagery is never far away from stone temples, which were often the site of blood sacrifice. In Mexico, the moon and sun temples are pyramidic forms, and the entire moon temple of Teotihuacan in the valley of Mexico was painted blood red.[24] As with the Egyptian, Mayan, and Chinese temples, Greek temples and related buildings were richly colored, the most prominent color being red. Sumerian doors were also painted red. The mountain-shaped moon temple at Ur was black at the bottom to signify the underworld, red in its main body for earth, and capped with a little blue hut for sky. A feature of a tall Chichén Itzá pyramid is that by a trick of architecture, a huge serpent appears to slide down the side of the great structure at dusk of the equinox.[25] Many Mayan temples have serpents depicted on or otherwise associated with them, as Asian temples have dragons.

In farming communities on rivers, the temple of orientation was also an early-warning flood system—an ark if ever there was one. This is believed to have been one use of the Great Pyramid, which marked the rising of the star Sothis, an event that preceded the Nile's yearly flood by two weeks—long enough for farmworkers to move to higher ground.[26] Three calendric measurements, lunar, solar and stellar, are incorporated into its dimensions. The pyramid is almost perfectly oriented to true north and incorporates a value for *pi* accurate to several decimals. It also incorporates the sacred triangle 3-4-5 and the formula $a^2 + b^2 = c^2$, "which were to make Pythagoras famous, and which Plato in his *Timaeus* claimed as the building blocks of the cosmos"[27]. The pyramid's angles and slopes display trigonometric values, and its shape uses the proportions of the "Golden Section." The top of the pyramid represents the North

Pole, and the base of it, the equator; each quadrant of its face equaled 90 degrees of earth surface. Thus a structure combining the triangle and the square was used to describe perfectly the half-globe of the Northern Hemisphere of the earth.[28]

Builders of the Great Pyramid knew the exact circumference of the planet and the precise length of the year. Peter Tompkins, an engineer who compiled centuries of the Great Pyramid's measurements, thinks they may also have known the mean length of the earth's orbit around the sun, the specific density of earth, the 26,000-year cycle of the equinoxes, the acceleration of gravity and the speed of light. Since only scraps of this information passed over to the West through the Greeks, it could not be rediscovered until modern engineers had emerged from the so-called Dark Ages of European village life. In 820 A.D., Abdullah Al Mamun, patron of science, battered into the Great Pyramid after being told by his network of intelligence agents (1,700 old women) that the structure contained celestial and terrestrial maps. When the maps could not be found, in disappointment, his men hacked the beautiful granite walls. Later, Westerners used explosives to gain entrance. Only recently have engineers understood that the pyramid itself is a set of measuring tools.[29]

The Great Pyramid, in conjunction with two smaller ones near it, produces sets of triangular shapes and shadows of triangular shapes that can fix exact locations from an area hundreds of miles around. Using only a plumb bob, a farmer could redefine land boundaries after the yearly flood had washed the markers away.

In the middle of the Great Pyramid, and many others, are small chambers. Surrounded by tons of limestone, these chambers typically are made of granite slabs. They are hut-shaped and hut-sized, with peaked roofs. They have long been thought to be tombs for kings, though no king's bodies have been found. The main chamber of the Great Pyramid is tiny compared to the massive structure, and it has an anteroom—as though to leave food and water for a royal menstruant secluded in the coffer within.[30]

The archetypal ancient city arose in Mesopotamia and was sustained by a complex economy based in farming, herding, and the exchange of crafts. It was often located near a river and often had a lunar temple at its center, and female-headed priesthoods, incorporating kingship as masculine parallel *r'tu*. The temple was a kind of ark, a material container for orientation to the earth and to rotating lights in the sky, for purifying rites of fire and water, and for seclusion of menstrual officiants. It housed statuary—replicas of the collective menstruant, or deities—and encompassed sanctuaries and burial grounds. It was also a repository for substances of *cosmetikos* such as myrrh, turmeric, ochre, meat and herb sacrifices, grains, beers and wines, and carefully worked metaformic minerals, gems, and wooden objects of the master craftsmen. In Sumer, some five thousand years ago, Inanna's "temple," a word meaning "storehouse," was depicted on seals as a reed hut, like little reed menstrual huts in use recently in rural countrysides of neighboring India, or the sacred *giparu* of the Babylonian creation myth.[31] Inanna's actual temples had by then become huge stone structures, with big eastern doors, the centers of all civilian life in the cities considered "hers."

Goddesses of later Greece would wear crowns shaped like walled cities in tribute to the female role of origination of the urban form. Successfully dependent on metaforms of grains, meats, and fruits, populations now began to swell, and to gather in close quarters around the temple storehouse. Writing, beginning around 3500 B.C.E. in the Sumerian temples as a method of keeping track of the storing and distribution of grain, soon included tablets of narrative creation stories. Western culture was there, poised at the edge of a world view distinctly different from those developed by wilderness, *cosmetikos* and narrative metaforms—the new mind would be based in materialist metaforms.

Chapter 15

Crossing the Abyss to Male Blood Power

I N considering materialism, we have seen that it is rooted in the menstrual metaforms of craftspeople. Increasingly dependent on agriculture and herding, as well as on the horticulture and irrigation that developed in Mesopotamia and ancient Eygpt, human culture began to break away from wilderness metaform. Instead narrative *logos* and materialist metaform began to transform whole river valleys of the earth into farms and villages, and then temple-centered cities, toward which the trade of crafts gravitated.

Our story thus far has begged the question of *why?* Why was the break with "mother earth" and Snake so complete? Why did Eve cast her serpent of female instruction to the ground, changing it from a central metaform back to simply a creature? What became, in the West, of the rich goddess heritage archaeologists have unearthed from our near-past? How is it that some indigenous peoples of the Americas retain a female-centered, snake-revering, blood-based, and earth-protective tradition lost to the Spaniards and other Europeans who overran their continents after 1492? What became of menarchal rites? How did menstruation come to be listed as a biological condition rather than the center of the human mind and spirit? And why is the modern approach to matter and to female origins so different from that of the Kogi, or even the ancient Sumerians, who lined in long processions to bring their baskets of figs and their prize lambs to the temples of Venus and the moon couple? Most important, what became of the teachings of female menstruants to human consciousness and culture? What became of female origin story? The answers to these questions help define what we modern people mean by "materialism." Materialism began as the manipulation of earth into crafts, but it continued as a full-blown philosophical stance toward the earth and femaleness itself.

Proponents of the theory that goddess-centered cultures of the Neolithic period achieved peaceful farming civilizations have done an excellent job in reconstructing, from archaeological evidence, the iconography of their central female metaforms. It has been postulated that women developed pottery, weaving, farming, and a protectiveness toward animals and nature. According to proponents of "goddess theory," during the Bronze Age, men suddenly stole the goddess culture from women, usurped its rites, and established male rule and male sky gods by force of arms. Marija Gimbutas argues that nomadic herders with less-developed culture swept into the farming villages of Old Europe and replaced its complexities with more violent, warring stances. Warfare and violence replaced peaceful Neolithic "goddess cultures" throughout the Middle East.[1] Before speculating how and why this happened, let's take a look at what mythology can tell us about "stealing," from a menstrual point of view.

Male Tradition of Thievery

The accumulation of forms and ideas spill out of women's seclusion rites and pass over to the male domain, where they become public, extended completions of the cosmogony of the whole people. This passage happens through several vehicles, among them, parallel menstrual rites that lead to hunting, blood sacrifice, ritual games, and warrior battles. Another example of crossover is shamanism, that special male apprenticeship, often of men who identify with

249

the female. The office of the Shaman expanded in complex farming societies into that of holy man, priest, chief, and also king, pharoah, and mikado.

A third method by which menstrual knowledge transfers to the men is through the office of the male thief. Because, I believe, the male is always one step removed from actual physical correspondence with the lunar cycle, and from other metaphoric tools of the menstrual and birth huts, he has developed an ingenious tradition of ritualized, ceremonially acknowledged "thievery" to acquire cultural paraphernalia for his own uses and to explain his own creativity in the context of "new" metaforms.

In my family the men bragged about getting away with cheating or stealing. Primarily this was linguistic theft, not theft in a legal sense. "Go steal some when your mother isn't looking," my father would say of my desire to have cherry pie before dinner. My mother never used the word thief about us. She "borrowed" my father's things, and she was embarrassed when he spoke of himself, as he often did, as a thief. He on the other hand, loved the whole idea, stroking his chin or moustache with pleasure as he told a thief story on himself or called another man a "horse thief." On those occasions when he accused my mother of stealing from him, his screwdriver for example, she was completely mortified, and retreated into herself, furious and full of denial.

Motives for a male tradition of thievery are implied in the testimony of Native Australians: "the women have everything, the blood, the baby, everything . . ."[2] Women, through the offices of seclusion and direct blood synchrony, collect essential principles and metaforms, and the men, if they can't get them otherwise, break in to get them. According to some traditions, bold men "opened a hole in the women's weaving house," or overran the women's living complex, or through some other effort, acquired some of the paraphernalia women had developed. That this requires breaking taboos to which the whole society has agreed for

250

as long as anyone can recall perhaps accounts for the acts being called "stealing." Or, more likely, the notion of "theft" holds in place the idea of "original owner."

Male traditions of thievery are found among many peoples. In some South American tribes, the men describe suddenly raiding the women's part of a village and stealing "their things," including string and a flattened stick with which the men made a noisy instrument, a bull-roarer, which they then used to frighten the women. A global mythic tradition of men or boys stealing women's clothing, especially the clothing women leave on the river bank while they bathe, has been suggested by folklorist Martha Beckwith as the theft of menstrual garments.[3] Unless the women gave some of theirs, menstrual blood for sorcery, healing, or magic could be acquired only by stealing. In the West, we might see a fragment of this tradition in college dormitory panty raids!

The male theft of fire, and the sun, is another theme common to myths across a variety of cultures. In a northern Asiatic tradition, Old Grandmother's grandson stole fire from her and burned down the world. Prometheus stole fire from the sun in Greece—from the protomoon, men got the red fire, like blood. In one African myth, the culture hero Mokele "steals" the sun when he goes up a river and discovers the place where the sun lives in a cave.[4] This act of differentiation of the sun surely means he "stole" it from the original protomoon of the female tradition.

The Dogon people of the Sudan have formalized the rite of male sun thievery. In their cosmogony the first blacksmith stole fire from the sun, and the tongs with which he accomplished the deed have been carefully reproduced, passed through the generations and tended as sacred objects. In Ogotemmêli's words, "the smith went stealing with his robber's crook. It was in the mouth of this stick that fire began. That was the smith's gift to the world. That is why the institution of ritual theft was started." Ogotemmêli describes every family head in Sanga as a ritual thief, and a ritual crook was hung in the Dogon "big house." The ritual thieves also conducted raids on small livestock, "which were then eaten in common ac-

251

cording to prescribed conditions."[5] Since in the Dogon system the sun exudes liquid (copper) and is in the female domain, the smith's heavenly sortie was to steal a piece of the older menstrual tradition. With fire, iron, and the arts of the smith, an independent male office of trade and craft was established and carefully integrated into the Dogon village.[6]

Raiding and stealing, always under specific rules, have primarily been men's work, part of men's story. In myths from China to South America, some male characters are thieves who take, not only the paraphernalia of women, but women themselves, queens renowned for their beauty and slaves from other tribes. In addition, they make off with fire, the sun, livestock, treasures, technologies. One effect of this was the accumulation of materials and ideas from many different places, combining and recombining to form mechanical arts and complex trades. Another was the dispersal of "women's stuff" and tribal arts, scattered out from the sacred huts into the secular world. Men, more often than women, have widely dispersed and recombined knowledge, craft, trade, and story.

Male Separation from the Queen of Heaven and Earth

About twenty-five hundred years ago, not long after myths began to be etched onto clay tablets, a male-centered tradition ran off with the narrative religion of the paired elements descending from Tiamat and Apsu, the Great Sea and the Great Abyss. The gender-balanced pantheons that had existed for many millennia were consolidated into a single male creation deity. This theft differs from my earlier examples in that the stories of men's theft of women's things retain these female origin stories intact: women continue to be credited, they remain central to the story, so the role of *r'tu* is retained. When monotheistic men "stole" written narratives of female origin stories, they left female creation out. This was far more than ceremonial "stealing"; it constituted a complete overthrow, which eventually suppressed the older female traditions and lost a great deal of the whole story.

252

As we have seen from the discussion of how people approached the manipulation of physical matter, "weap-mon" was transformed into "crafts-mon." But the traders and artisans of ancient cities were just as immersed in the *r'tu* of the goddess-based religion as their fellow hunters, warriors, and farmers. But in at least one area of the world, as recorded in the mythology of Mesopotamia, men took another step, an independent step—they separated their identities and their sense of purpose from women, and from the feminine principle of menstrual *r'tu*.

The earliest account of "male separation" from the essential lunar tradition is in the myth of Gilgamesh, who we recall was a historic king of a Sumerian city around 2600 B.C.E. In the myth, "The One Who Looked into the Abyss," he faces off with the Queen of Heaven and Earth, Inanna/Ishtar. "Marry me," she says, "and I will give you anything you want." But his answer is a surprise. In effect he says, since you have everything in the world to offer, what could I possibly bring to such a match? And he then lists her six earlier suitors, beginning with the bull god Dumuzi, whose sacrificial death she annually mourns. He names the animal forms and sad plight of her other lovers: bird, lion, wolf, stallion, frog. Gilgamesh is saying that he refuses to become a wilderness metaform! And he refuses to enter a relationship of either sacrifice or dependency with her. Unlike his predecessors, he spurns marriage with the metaformic goddess because, he says, he wants to remain a mortal man.

The entire myth of this rebellious king centers on the establishment of a germinal male-centered stance toward wilderness, identity, paternity, and the goddess religion. Enraged by his dismissal of her, Inanna/Ishtar sends a bull to kill him. The king and his companion, Enkidu, the "wild man," kill the bull instead, tricking the gods. The institution of the bullfight thus substitutes the sacrifice of the bull for the royal victim. As followers of the sun deity, who is Inanna/Isthar's brother, Utu, the two men go into the forest of sacred cedars, kill the guardian spirit, and cut the tabooed red-barked trees. They let the sun shine directly on the earth. For their

253

crime against *r'tu,* Enkidu is condemned by a pantheon of con-
cerned deities, who send him a fatal illness. (This part of the myth
might be read as a description of the annihilation of indigenous
peoples all over the earth by diseases borne by urban civilizations,
a process that has not yet been stopped.)

Unable to sit still for the duration of the old funeral practices,
Gilgamesh undertakes a journey to find the spirit of Enkidu, to ask
if immortality exists. "I sat by him until a worm fell out of his
nose," he laments. What is called into question here is the fundamental lunar story of cycles, of rebirth and reincarnation. When
Gilgamesh finally does find Enkidu, his friend is merely a ghostly
voice speaking from the underworld: "The flesh you loved to
touch" has rotted away, he reports. Immortality through reincarnation, the cyclic system taught by the temple priestesses, is false.
The only immortality for man, Enkidu says, lies with material
reproduction of male progeny. He lists a new sequence of "eternal
life": the man with one son does fairly well, the man with two does
a little better, and so on, until the man with seven sons, who does
the best of all—and whose memory lives on in the honoring his
sons give his name. The myth ends here, in a new doctrine of paternity and of physical reproduction as the only guarantee of a
place in the world ruled by the sun god, "a place in the sun."

Perhaps it was the differentiation and close study of the habits of
the sun that led to a crisis of faith in the lunar narratives, especially
in the Mesopotamian area, where—unlike many other places—the
sun was designated male and associated with paternity. The lunar
menstrual ritual passed over to Utu's sister, Inanna, the deified
planet Venus, whose poets gave her a character both fierce and
tender to carry the massive weight of the menstrual tradition. The
new perspective that the sun, being male, did not menstruate, did
not have a three-day darkness every month, left the way open for a
new story to emerge. At the same time, the development of planting
by seed instead of cuttings and a new emphasis on manufacturing
through pottery and crafts would have given physical reproduction
a new emphasis. The herding arts that had replaced human sacri-

254

fice also externalized paternity, as herders inevitably noticed the effects of breeding certain rams and bulls with certain ewes and cows.[7] Gradually, in the ancient Near East, paternity became the object of human "study" and the focus of its religious doctrines. Father gods had held prominent positions in the sky, sea, and even the earth in many religious myths, but always in conjunction with female deities. But the new father god, the god of Abraham, was different from these, and different even from the monotheistic sun god of Ahkenaton in Egypt. Though the pharaoh tried to establish a single deity in the form of the sun, and many other peoples in the Northern Hemisphere also worshiped the sun, the new religion could not use old wilderness metaforms to create a unified creator deity. The monotheistic god could not be anthropomorphically attached to a planet, star, or other natural formation and still be the All-being who oversaw a universe that—thanks to the measurements and observations of temple astronomers—was rapidly expanding in size. The very success of the sciences of the goddess priesthoods and the pervasiveness of earth as menstrual Mother eventually disenfranchised them. The All-god, needing new parameters of description, crossed over to a new male tradition—one that did not use wilderness or *cosmetikos* metaforms to describe him. Once again, the metaform extended by crossing the Great Abyss of changing consciousness.

Born as he was in a world saturated with goddess ritual and goddess iconography, the All-father deity had to be singular and jealous to be truly monotheistic. He also had to take many of the characteristics of the goddesses before him, as there were no other terms for "greatest" deity. The greatest deity was the one who had the full weight of menstrual creation tradition behind it. The priests and priestesses who founded the religion of Yahweh therefore endowed him with some of the character of older gods—especially elements of Enki and Inanna—but only enough to establish him as Great and to continue his definition as a god of paternity, a god who promises polygamous Abraham success with his "seed," his progeny. Yahweh thus has Inanna's title of "Great" but not her *cosmetikos.* He has a throne and the Flood myth, and like her he rules "heaven and earth," but he has lost the underworld and the older sister Ereshkigal and the art of giving birth. He is "eternal" and does not go through menstrual cycles or rebirth as Inanna did. He was her ferocity, to protect his people, to slay his enemies, to bring down mountains, but he does not have her sacred marriage or her rampant sexuality. Nor does he have the homosexual priest-hood that marched in her New Year's procession or the sacred whores who officiated in her temples.

To account for these missing elements—which of course did not go away, since they are central to human culture—a new character was invented: Satan.[8] All the menstrual characteristics of creation/decreation that could not be molded into Yahweh's fatherness were gradually, over the centuries, consigned to "the evil shade" and the realm of "sin," a word related to the moon. As he developed through medieval times, Satan's red color, three-pronged fork, se-ductive sexual qualities, his embodiments as serpent, goat, black dog, and dragon all speak eloquently to the inversion of the essen-tial metaform. As the paternal religions sharpened their definitions, menstrual *r'tu* was increasingly suppressed, and Satan grew in di-mension as a character outside of the Father's realm—cast away, blamed, and avoided.

Though the sun could not be sustained as the "Great" deity of Western civilization, one of the key elements of the paternal reli-gion's focus was its identification with light, especially with light's ability to cleanse and complete. During the centuries following the fall of Rome, all across the Euroasian continent, both the power of enlightenment and the power of light to "wash" one "clean of sin" attached to male deities. The Christian god extended paternity one step by being the Son of the (slightly) older Father, but he also was given the menstrual traditions of the Mother. In a new Descent myth, the bleeding Son was hung on a peg-tree-cross, to die for three lunar days before a glorious resurrection—just as Inanna had before him. In the Christian mechanism of forgiveness, both wrongdoings and debts were declared cleansed, washed away, by a simple change of inner feeling toward the wrongdoer and the verbal statement, "I forgive you." In secular materialist terms, "The creditor forgives this debt." Increasingly, male blood was considered "clean" and generative, while female blood was only "unclean" and destructive. Male ritual was associated with creation, while menstrual creation was forgotten and suppressed.

Herding, Disease, and Menstrual Shame

In the goddess-based religions, nonreproductive sexuality had been a lush part of *r'tu*. It promoted visions and physical health in Chinese and Indian Tantric traditions, and it was also understood to bring rain, to make the crops grow, to help the herds increase, and generally to enhance the well-being and fertility of the countryside surrounding the temple complexes. In the new male-centered laws, nonreproductive and unmarried sex were severely restricted, to ensure exact paternity. The principles used in herding were applied to human reproduction. This necessitated controlling sexuality, especially of the mother, and of banning—and eventually satanizing—all sex that did not lead to reproduction. The arts of lovemaking and control of reproduction, carefully tended by sacred prostitutes in temple rites and by village midwives, disappeared. Some Christian sects and later monastic orders undertook celibacy for long periods of time and with mixed success, but with the aim of neutralizing the female influence while continuing the essential church and temple rites. The genders would blend, according to this ideal, and both would become the clean, pure male.[9]

The factors leading to this extraordinary crossover from the rich female-centered pantheons that established urban and farm life to the "seminal" and "conceptual" ideology of the male All-god can only be guessed. But it is clear that a shift in blood sacrifice was one such factor. The god of Abraham had replaced human sacrifice with animal sacrifice, and gradually the herdsman's "mentality"—a concern with paternal line, with offspring—became more completely integrated into the worlds of farmers and craftsmen. And perhaps the more successfully human sacrifice was replaced, the guiltier menstruation itself became. In Genesis, the earth is described as "thirsty for blood." The fields of farmers from the Mediterranean to the Indian Ocean, and beyond, were saturated with human blood. Not only agriculture but evidently even crafts required ritual use of blood: "The Goddess was worshipped as a Potter in the Jewish temple, where she received 'thirty pieces of silver' as the price of a sacrificial victim (Zechariah 11:13). She owned the Field of Blood, Aceldama, where clay was moistened with the blood of victims so bought. Judas, who allegedly sold Jesus for this same price, was himself another victim of the potter. In the Potter's Field he was either hanged (Matthew 27:5) or disemboweled (Acts 1:18), suggesting that the Potter was none other than the Goddess who both created and destroyed." [10]

But craftspeople themselves had helped to end certain forms of human sacrifice by their arts. In India, the r'tu of sacrifice was acted out by using a wooden statue of the central female metaform, taking the statue completely apart, lying it down in seclusion for a specified period of time, and then reassembling and "washing" it with a new coat of paint. In earlier times, the fields of the same area had been littered with human parts. [11]

It seems only logical to assume that as human sacrifice, especially of one's relatives and of children, was completely replaced by the "blood-offering" of statues and herd animals—and later barley-cakes and flowers—shame would follow from what the people had formerly done. [12] Menstruation, being at the heart of r'tu, would take the full brunt of blame, as it did for incest-consciousness and death-consciousness in other cultures and eras. Even so this scenario does not adequately explain the deep submergence of menstruation and the vulva to the point of utter unspeakability— sustained, even in my family in the 1950s, some one to two thousand years after the last of my north European ancestors would have taken the eldest son or youngest daughter to the drought-starved fields and used their blood to solicit rain.

A second idea occurs to me as a possible explanation for the depth of menstrual shame. Recently, historians have acknowledged the role of disease in the conquest of the North and South American continents, first by the Spanish, and then the French and English—opening the way for waves of settlers and immigrants from every nation on earth. It is now estimated that 95 percent of the indigenous peoples perished of diseases brought from the European continent, most of them within a few decades of contact in 1492.[13] All of these diseases had been introduced over millennia into human populations on the Euroasian continent by their close contact with the herding animals they had brought under domestication species by species. The bacilli, harmless while living in the animals, mutated in the human body, producing virulent strains of highly communicable illness, to which Europeans, because of repeated exposure, were less susceptible.

But the populations of the Americas and places like the Hawaiian Islands, which also lost most of its peoples to illness, had domesticated very few animals—on the south American continent, only the llama, muscovy duck, and guinea pig, and further north, only the turkey. The people had no defenses whatsoever against the sudden exposure to so many bacilli, especially smallpox, the most devastating of many dreadful diseases.

This was one of the cruelest paradoxes of menstrual *r'tu* and culture: that the development of herding economies, which helped to replace the practice of human sacrifice, was responsible, from 1492 through the present, for the greatest die-off of humans and of entire cultures in any recorded or remembered history.[14] Perhaps, because no one had any other explanation, the blame for the catastrophe fell on the deities of the older religions—the great snake goddesses and jaguar gods, the sun, moon, and planet deities of the Mayans and Aztecs. The relative immunity of the conquerors seemed an act of divine judgment, and it gave their paternal god

259

incredible power. Horrified and conscientious native shamans and priests sometimes urged their people to become Christians to save them from the plagues. The royalty of the Hawaiian Islands and other native leaderships led the way to the new male-centered religion, though of course Christian priests could not stop the dying either. Only immunization would accomplish that, and not fully, and not until the twentieth century.

Might it not be possible that similar plagues killed people in the Middle East and Europe as the herding-based paternal religions first began to spread? Marija Gimbutas describes the goddess-worshiping culture of Neolithic Europe, whose rich settlements were suddenly replaced by simpler horse-based patriarchal herders, whose invasions virtually erased the older civilizations.[15] Perhaps smallpox was the more virulent culprit there as well—the pestilence that came in the wake of the nomadic peoples would have strengthened belief in the "power" of the masculine deity to "punish" unbelievers.

As farming and herding allowed population densities to rise, plagues began to appear, and they are recorded in the mythology of Mesopotamia, where the earliest known cities developed: At Babylon, the Gilgamesh Flood myth specifies plague as one of mankind's four ills; an illness sent by avenging gods kills Enkidu, the wilderness man; and plague is in Egypt before the writing of Exodus. Yahweh, like Inanna before him, is a deity who brings illness at will, and he does so specifically to punish those who are not faithful to his paternal tenets. The new male doctrine, in short, used natural disasters to frighten people and promote itself.

Of the fatal diseases that sweep human populations, smallpox was one of the deadliest, and the red dots typical of the disease may have enhanced its association with the menstrual power of annihilation. In India, one of Kali's titles is "goddess of smallpox"—and Kali, we recall, is completely connected to the dark menstrual moon. Two goddesses, sisters of course, tended by artisans in a village in rural India, are named for illnesses: "Prayers are then offered to the goddesses asking that the village be free from cholera and smallpox, for Durgamava is believed to preside over and cause cholera, while Dayamava is the presiding deity of smallpox."[16]

It is thus very possible that the ancient goddess of menstruation, however she was imagined, was believed to have sent the most crushing of the plagues of humankind and that this intensified the fear, punishment, and shame associated with menstruation, helping to establish the male-based religions of "light." Perhaps a series of plagues lies behind both the spread of Christianity into pagan Europe and the waves of witch trials that followed the bubonic plague, which killed one out of three Europeans in the fourteenth and fifteenth centuries. That the fears about these mostly poor and old women were tied to old menstrual taboos is clear. They were believed to cause illness from a distance, with the gaze of the Evil Eye. They were identified as "real" witches by their association with old wilderness metaforms: one woman "vomited eels"; others "evacuated snakes"; some turned into birds, goats, or dogs. In Norway, witches were thought to cause storms by turning into geese or by whistling. Catholic theologians held that Satan could turn men into wolves, but that women were the greatest evil, spreading illness with a gaze, rotting men's bodies, deserving of shame simply for being women.[17] Though the Inquisition was politically motivated and served the avaricious male leadership to seize property and authority from traditional women healers and diviners, there is no doubt that in times of stress European peasants and townspeople, Catholic and Protestant alike, were genuinely frightened of anyone believed to have the old menstrual powers. In the absence of the germ theory of disease and other mechanics of natural cause and effect, people blamed the symptoms of illness, epilepsy, and all manner of other disasters, on the same power they had always held responsible: menstruation. But now they called the metaform "Satan," and they imputed evil motives not only to the menstruant but to their neighbors and to whole groups of people with older (and more menstrually based) traditions—Jews, gypsies, homosexuals, and prostitutes. They were fearful of people with darker or redder physical characteristics. But in particular the Evil

Eye was imputed to old women, who were believed to retain their menstrual blood so that it flowed through their veins following menopause![18]

The menstrual gaze was imagined as Satan-directed "possession," which could be cured simply by something as male as the symbol of the phallus.[19] The Evil Eye was called "fascination" and could be counteracted with the male "fasces," a bundle of phallic sticks—hence fascism's association with the "fire of male cleansing." The Evil Eye and its subjective responsibility could be replaced through spoken prayer and charms invoking "God's Eye," the Eye outside the woman, the Eye from above.

The Rise of Clean Male Light

Gradually, from Catholicism and Greek orthodoxy through the Protestant reform movements, Christianity stripped itself of all but the most narrative approach to blood ritual. In the English, German, and Swedish Protestantism of my grandmothers, women not only were kept away from the sacred ritual, they also wore only the slightest *cosmetikos*. The old *cosmetikos* of slashing of the skin and tatooing had been forbidden since the writing of the laws of Leviticus, but these women took austerity much further. They held their faces very still, engaged in no public mourning, kept their food as white as possible, never threw plates, did not dance or move their pelvises—as though they ordered their world through the degree of stillness and paleness they could maintain in the face of any adversity. They expressed themselves instead with small collections of miniature crafts, kept in glass cupboards and carefully displayed and dusted. (One of the signs of possession by "Satan," the Inquisition taught, was expression of enthusiasm.) And no mention of menstruation, no memory of its connection to religion and female origins of culture, no use of the Jewish menstrual bath and celebration of sexuality, no calling in of the Shekinah, no statues showing Christ's blood running down his side, no Madonna standing on her crescent moon and her snake. The Sabbath of separation had become associated solely with the clean male light, the Son/Sun of Sunday. Even one's disposition was supposed to be relentlessly "sunny"—no "dark" underworld feelings. The old office of female mourner lost its blood-slashed face and vulva, lost its wailing and its black veil, and then among my people, vanished.[20]

No secret violent tempers my mother ever exerted on her children can be discussed with her. She acts as though they never happened. If I press her with an example, she speaks vaguely of "past mistakes," but never acknowledges details. As a female child under my mother's roof, I could not drink, curse, talk about sex or death, whistle, dance, talk with my hands, yawn without covering my mouth, sleep past 7:00 A.M., or be overly enthusiastic on any subject. I could not discuss blood or any violence. When I was very young, up to about age eight, I had to stand silently for an hour or two in the corner of the living room, facing the wall like a menstruant of old, if I broke a minor rule. (But menstruants had stood facing the wall for weeks, not hours.)

My mother's house rules were not as rigid as those under my Swedish grandmother's roof, which my sister tells me forbade girls to leave the house on Sunday, even to go into the yard, constraining them to sit still all day, carefully dressed from top to bottom in white.

During much of the era of the patriarchal gods, women have virtually been in seclusion, subduing the red dragon power equated, through the old narratives, with the most drastic evils to befall humankind. Through its denial of physicality, especially female physicality, the Christian religion has led humanity squarely into the middle of the materialist metaform.

Materialism, as I have imagined, began with crafts and architecture as a means of ordering the menstrual world, manipulating minerals and clay as the earth's blood and flesh. "Goods," processed metaformic objects, were hauled on ships imagined as vulvas of the goddess—hence the female figures and dragon's heads

263

on ship bows, and the amazing amount of menstrual taboo associated with sailing and fishing. But as the goods themselves became
central metaforms for success, the materials of the earth became
"products," just as did the infant materials of the womb. Birth became "labor," a work that "produced" a "product," and human
beings came to be traded and designated slave or owner. These
elements combined into the philosophy of materialism, which sees
the earth from "outside" rather than from "within" or "as part of"
its processes. The male god was increasingly identified with the
purifying element, light, while the feminine remained tied to the
old menstrual definitions of the earth, now shamed and defiled
with illness and blood, nonpaternal sex, and naked wilderness.

The shift to a single male deity directed human consciousness
toward a state of objectification. The new male perspective, allied
with the cleansing fire of the sun and based in menstrual crafts that
processed the "female" substance of earth, denied all subjectivity,
intuition, meditation, and the female arts of sexual connection and
r'tu. The new perspective was completely "off the earth," not the
few yards of the menstruant hanging in her hammock, but miles
high on a heavenly throne. Whereas in former times, only menstrual blood itself and a few metaforms had been considered per-
manently unclean, the very substance of the earth—all matter—
came to be seen as polluted. Earth's abundance was valued only if
it could be cooked, burned, baked, boiled, shaved, painted, covered, tamed, dressed—processed into a product, suitable for trade.
Deity now overlooked the earth; it was no longer within the earth.
This separated the human psyche from the earth's psyche, stripping
the natural world of sacredness, intelligence, or creative interaction
with humankind.

Because the female origin stories were suppressed by written narratives of male origin stories, the goddess tradition was lost. Materialism led people to trade crafts with more and more frenzy and
without remembering why. By 1492, a Europe terrified by plague
and witchcraft sent Columbus and other explorers to gather protective cosmetikos from other peoples—gold to line the churches,

spices to color and flavor food and make it more "healthful," and herbs, even tobacco, as health aids.

Perhaps, as the earth itself was treated more and more as a menstrual substance and "taken over by Satan," *r'tu* lost its power and humankind could no longer protect themselves by their own actions, by adherence to ritual law. Salvation could only come from above—from light, from grace. In the Christian West, this view was nevertheless sustained by images of the purifying "blood of Christ," which "washes," "redeems," "forgives," and "saves." But the earth was no longer seen as alive or enspirited. In materialist metaformic terms, raw matter was inert and defiling, woman was guilty of evoking its "sins," and man was alone on its broad dangerous surface, looking off the earth, seeking light and eternity.

Ages of Light versus Dark

The values underlying social categories based on differentiating the sun from the earth are completely embedded in language. "Lower" is connected to earthy, and menstrual earth is the source of ideas like soiled, crude, cloddish, inert, mucky. Dirt is considered unclean and unhealthy. Parts of the earth are equated in common speech with disliked female body parts and sexual behavior: slime, bog, tangle, deep, dark, damp, smelly. Elements connected to the older, prematerialist cultures have been "cast away" in the developing male doctrine, so the metaformic creatures that gave us our minds to begin with are often particularly persecuted—the creatures who live close to the earth and crawl and the predators that represent "death." Ideas of "good" and "bad" are applied to classes of people, animals, and portions of the earth as well—as though it does not all work together, as though death, menstruation, and the earth itself are our enemies. Good qualities are associated with the sky—hence "upper" and "superior" are desirable, "lower" and "inferior" are not. Light is considered cleansing, intelligent, healthy; intelligence is brilliance, brightness; health glows; inspiration is a spark that lights a fire.

All the negativity associated with disease and menstrual destruction is applied, through speech, to entire groups of people. We could say that the negative menstrual-based associations which are connected to racism, anti-Semitism, classism, sexism, homophobia, and related caste systems are all applied, not only to people, but also to the earth and its "raw" life forms. This can only accelerate the materialist zeal to drain swamps, cover over wetlands, strip trees or plant them in military rows for the purpose of "producing" an "orderly" world. (But the more we "produce" the earth, and the more one group persecutes another, the more disorder threatens to engulf us).

These materialist beliefs could be called *necroforms*—metaforms that have not only grown out of sync with the greater knowledge of science and religion alike, but that actively work against the survival of the ecosystem. They are on the same level as belief that disease is caused by the menstruant's "evil-eyed gaze." We are in grave danger and put the planet in grave danger as long as we continue to use necroforms. They are illogical separations that shred the social fabric of nations and the web of life on earth.

Male Seclusion and Male Science

In the centuries after Christianity established itself in Europe, the church began to exclude women from positions of religious power. Especially in the twelfth century, when the office of abbess had lost its former authority, religious orders became institutions of male seclusion. The word "monk" means separate, alone. Many of the orders stressed years of isolation, simple meals, fasting, holding severe positions for days on end—similar to the disciplines of menstrual *r'tu*. However, the men distanced themselves from the feminine by criticizing the arts of women. Augustine, for instance, deplored the seductive habit women had of lowering their eyes, and looking down at the ground. All humans were evil, but women were especially susceptible to Satan's wiles. (And given that Satan's qualities were taken directly from the most ancient menstrual rites, misogynist theologians like Augustine were accurate in their assessment—as far as it went.)

The institutions of male seclusion created a kind of "seminal mind," by taking control of origin story, seizing control of written biblical narrative, and forbidding the rituals, pageants, and other enactments that carried the female tradition in nonverbal form. In the monasteries, "monkish scientists" who spoke only to other men developed rationalism and other fundamentals of modern science as methods of further understanding God. "At the outset . . . the culture of science was the culture of the ecclesiastical academy and, hence, a world without women. . . . Western science first took root in an exclusively male—and celibate, homosocial, and misogynous—culture, all the more so because a great many of its early practitioners belonged also to the ascetic mendicant orders."[21]

For several centuries, the university system developed as a cloistered society of men who identified deity as a light from above, "off the earth." In Descartes's mechanistic view, only God was living. Early scientists from Copernicus to Newton searched for a male creation deity as Absolute Being, unchanging, noncyclic. For Kepler, the sun was the "purest light," worthy to be the home of God. Newton thought that atoms were unchangeable building blocks ruled by immutable mathematical laws. Others believed that mathematical patterns proved a fixed creative principle that could be comprehended by (European) man, and *through him* by women and others designated "inferior" status. In their flight from earth and the body, men succeeded in lifting human consciousness out of the subjective matrix of older metaforms into a new position: the nonintuitive view of matter, from off its surface.[22] Materialism, one might say, is identification with light, and with the *point of view* of light, especially as it examines surfaces. And as was true of earlier seclusions, the contents of monkish cells and science libraries spilled out into the secular world, impelled by the democratic ideal of allowing everyone who desires it to have a university education.

267

Among other discoveries of this external light—based science are the idea that nature has laws of its own, independent of human actions, and the germ theory of disease, which mostly has laid to rest witch-hunting doctrines of illness. Even so, many people retain deep shame about certain diseases. That AIDS is related to both sex and blood has made education about its causes very difficult. The shame and silence taboo and the pariah status of HIV positive people, lead to secrecy and greater risk of the disease's spread. Not only AIDS but all genital diseases carry the old menstrual stigma. In my mother's generation, it was also cancer (she cannot speak the word), and in her mother's generation tuberculosis, which displays blood and which killed my mother's father. Recently my mother told me that when she was born in Kansas in 1903, the doctor who delivered her had arrived fresh from a case of smallpox, infecting her. "They didn't know much about what caused such things in those days," she said. "I recovered, but I was always the smallest person in any crowd." She looked sad then, so that I wondered how many years of shame she had lived with, before the germ theory of disease lifted the veil of judgment and fear.

Though the male "theft" of goddess worship oppressed women, it also has gradually freed us from older bonds, from the phenomenal but also enslaving responsibility of having created everything, of having to hold everything in place, of having the power to destroy everything with a gaze, a touch, or a breath of air whistling through the lips. The sciences in the age of light lead us out of many of our older shames and inaccurate beliefs. But they did so at the price of female origin story. Science, that is, modern society, uses male origin story to explain itself, giving humans only a partial story with which to cope with our complex planet. Origin stories are never only about the past; they always affect how we act in the present. Young people entering the university system without knowing its history as a male-developed institution may imagine they are entering halls where "all knowledge" resides. They may, like me, drop out of school to search for more real truths. Worst of all, men imagine they must take responsibility for everything, their tradition is believed to be the root of human culture, and we are taught to believe we have no choice but to follow them.

War Metaforms

Under the influence of male origin story, war has replaced menstruation as the primary cause of mayhem, but war is simply an extension of old warrior games of ritual sacrifice—a parallel menstrual practice. Originating as sacrificial games played between villages or as mythic bouts with the powers of wilderness, warrior traditions burst out as armies of conquest when city-states battled each other's metaforms with warriors dressed as jaguars, wolves, and predatory birds.

Like menstruants and hunters, warriors abstained from sex, and they endured parallel menstrual disciplines—keeping silence, altering their diets, removing their hair, covering their heads, painting and slashing their bodies, and wearing animal metaforms of horns, quills, feathers and skins related to the origin stories of their peoples. Sometimes they wore veils. The medieval European king went out on the field with his armies as he had gone hunting, carried in a covered litter. When warriors returned to their village, they underwent purification rites, separation, steaming and bathing, fasting, and other restrictions to remove the menstrual stigma of the "blood on their hands."

War is primarily for the socializing of young men. In urban-based cultures of the past, war was an extension of ritual games in which "the gods like it better if some of us die."[23] That war pits the warrior against his own fear is evident from battles Celtic warriors once fought *against the waves of the sea*.[24] They waded out, heavy swords in hand, and sliced at waves (Tiamat's great walls of water) until their feet went out from under them and they either drowned or made it back to the beach. They were, perhaps, cutting the dragon in half. Celtic warriors also had many bloody confrontations with each other, keeping blood feuds going among their clans for centuries on end, a practice controlled only by Christian

269

intervention. Male Celtic warriors retained old menstrual beliefs. For instance, if a barefoot woman crossed the road in front of their band, they caught her and extracted blood from her forehead to keep from being "cursed" by her crossing.[25]

War took on economic motive in the cultures of materialism, which value the paraphernalia of *cosmetikos* without regard for its connection to any local *r'tu,* seeing wilderness as "raw material" to be converted into products. War accelerates the dispersal and recombination of elements in new ways. Modern war acclimates people to advances in technology, by placing soldiers and civilians alike under intense stress. Whether the latest technology is a shift from spears to bows, arrows to bullets, guns to gasses and chemicals, sharp ears to radar, horses to tanks, tanks to helicopters, mortar rockets to atomic explosives, much of what is developed in a war later comes home into civilian life, for good and ill.

The Chinese invented gunpowder, wrapping it in red paper and setting it afire to fight evil spirits at New Year's—the menarche of the year. Gunpowder was taken over by the masculine tradition of the West, and the gun has been associated with the penis ever since Freud defined it as a universal symbol of the masculine unconscious. But in menstrual logic, the gun is a metaform. Like the penis in defloration, it has the ability to induce bleeding. The Tiwi, we recall, believed that coitus led to the onset of menstruation, and early Native Americans believed that stepping over arrows or bows could cause a woman to begin her period. The metaformic power of these penile weapons comes from their association with blood, not semen.

In the West, origin stories are often based in war and the belief that male aggression first pushed primates into humanity. These ideas are put forth by scientists as well as by pop television shows. Male-centered myths begin by assigning an invention to a particular form of warfare—the wheel, for instance, is commonly believed to have been developed for war chariots. But as we have seen, early wheels were attached to the ox-carts that pulled Hera on her path between seclusion and the river, and between the river and her marriage on the mountain to the god of light. Similar carts were found in an excavation of a mass grave of red-dressed priestesses at Ur, and perhaps belonged to the moon goddess Ningal or her daughter Inanna. War chariots were a brief flash of human history, not usable without roads. And the earliest roads—*la via*, "the way"—were those of the path of the moon goddess and the moon god as they were dragged in procession through ancient cities. Not until Rome did roads have military importance. And even in the Roman army, menstrual imagery was never far from the battlefield—rose petals were strewn under Roman war chariots, as today paper petals are thrown over returning generals in processions.

Armies today still use *cosmetikos* in their rituals, as in the term dress-right-dress, meaning to line troops up straight. They also use humiliation, sleep deprivation, severe body postures, seclusion, silence taboos, and other methods of discipline to instill self-control in "raw" recruits, who are cooked into soldiers after being "dressed down" by tough-mouthed sergeants. White gloves are used in inspections to look for "dirt," but the warriors are no longer conscious of the menstruant who lay still in long white gloves, prohibited from touching her all-powerful blood.

Since the bombing of Hiroshima and Nagasaki, we have lived with the probability of annihilation, if not through atomic explosions then surely through the degeneration of the world environment by the stockpiling and dispersal of men's light-based weapons. Albert Einstein, after helping to develop the nuclear bomb, warned that men cannot solve the problems they have created in the twentieth century with the technology of the twentieth century. As poet Audre Lorde said, "For the master's tools will never dismantle the master's house."[26]

But blood, not war, is the central organizing principle of human culture. What tools can we use, then? Does women's *r'tu* have the answers?

Chapter 16

■■■■■■■■■■■■■■■■■■

The Way and the Way Back

After my father died, my mother gave away almost everything that was his—all his tools and his woodcarvings of pirates and sea captains, his crafts, his letters and clothes, some of the furniture he had made, and of course all his rifles and pistols. She hadn't liked her marriage, she said—which hurt me at first, until I tried to see it from her point of view. I remembered his know-it-all attitudes and his browbeating. But, she told me secretly, he "comes to visit" her sometimes, sitting in the overstuffed chair across from hers. From this I know she loved some essence of the man, if not the relationship they enacted in sixty years of sharing the same bed.

To replace his stuff, which like his stories had dominated their space, she has gathered around her all kinds of handicrafts, made primarily by women—her friends and relatives, her daughter (my sister) and granddaughters. Most of these objects are fabric weavings—shawls, wooly wall hangings, doilies, a blue sunbonnet. Her new things are colorful, cheerful, friendly.

As I prepare to visit her for Christmas, she writes that she wants roses, long-stemmed white silk roses with one or two green leaves. I understand immediately why she wants white roses. She wants innocence, as she prepares for death. When I arrive with the roses, I find she is no longer angry with my father. "Did you like him?" she asks, and I tell her, "We were very close." Recently, she confides, as she stared at a landscape picture on the wall, it began to glow and delivered a message to her, a single word: "Clean."

Menstrual Creation Principles

I think of the ancestress once again, sitting still in her shed, holding back the Flood with her bowls and straws. I recall how she entrained her consciousness with her sisters' bleeding, with the proto-moon, with dogs, jackal, and the black leopard; with the red ant mound and with Snake; with Great Tiamat the sea and with earth's fresh waterways; with the "blood" of red meat and with red fire; with plant sap, roots, fruits, grains, and flowers; with the bloody geometric strings of cat's cradle and the veins of precious minerals; and with the sun and planets and the razor Pleiades. When we sit on a chair, lift a fork, cook a meal, work a mathematical formula, use a triangle, name a planet, we are using products of menstrual origin. The menstrual mind underlies all that we are. It is the matrix, and it is always with us, no matter how we hide ourselves away from it.

Modern women are reemerging into public life from a long seclusion. Menstruation, too, is emerging as a subject "cleansed" of its former stigmas and powers. Absolved of its earlier connection to sin and danger, its old taboos are dismissed as superstitions or cataloged in anthropological terms. Menstruation is now described medically, a part of feminine hygiene (from Hygiea, another name for Athena the wise). Science understands menstruation as a hormonally controlled cycle with a well-defined place in reproduction. In addition, and congruently, the twentieth century has absorbed fully the biological comprehension of conception, from the gathering of racing sperms in their testicular sac to the arrival of the singular hero in the fallopian tube after a journey rivaling that of Odysseus. The winning bridegroom burrows into the wall of egg to join his spiral of coded information with hers. Paternity can now be established by technology, and has thus fulfilled its long journey to establish its place in creation.

It is time to move into the next cycle. Materialism is not the last Word. In menstrual theory, interactions among body, mind, spirit, and culture create "the human mind." The creation principles of menstrual theory seem to me to fall into two groups of triads:

273

(1) *Separation* is elemental, splitting off as a method of differentiating from the mass, and using taboos to regulate boundaries of behavior and establish categories. The natural phenomenon of entrainment of the inner menstrual cycle with the outer lunar cycle is a gift of nature that allowed ancestral females to comprehend patterns of synchrony, beginning with the idea that all blood is menstrual blood. From the equating of one kind of blood with another, the ancestors developed metaforms, the second principle of creation. (2) *Metaforms* are the external menstrual measurements with which humans extended their idea of synchrony to such natural forms as red ochre and blood-smeared predatory animals and vaginal snakes. By using metaform, the women could return from separation and instruct others, the third principle of creation. (3) *Instruction* taught and displayed ideas to the nonmenstruating members of their families, who also used metaforms to reflect their comprehensions.

Upon these three rest another triad, which greatly extend them. Derived from the course of the menstruant as she imitated the cycles of the moon, sacred story, or *hieros logos,* gave us menstrual logic. (4) *Menstrual logic* is the narrative plot that extended the human mind out in a net that encompassed all manner of cycles, and that continues to do so as scientists find patterns in biorhythms, geology, economic cycles, and radiowaves from distant galaxies.

The first four creation principles alone would have produced a static, small world without the effects of the last two, substitution and crossing, which have enabled huge social shifts. (5) The *substitution* of one metaform for another is represented in the Karok myth of how salmon was brought to the people. The two sisters break the salmon taboo they have placed on their people, and usher in a new age for their tribe, after Coyote eats red alder wood and calls it "salmon." The substitution of one metaform for another (wood for fish) effects a social change. The carpenters of village India substituted wooden figures for human victims, as did the craftsmen of gold and clay figurines. And this substitution—which

274

has to be a metaformic transformation deeply believed by the people—enabled their societies to change. The pretend murder of carefully tended and well-loved statues took the place of religious ritual murder. The carpenters, smiths, and other craftspeople successfully "tricked" the deep fear of drought, flood, and famine that everywhere has haunted farming people, redirecting this powerful emotion along a more benign path. This "tricking of the gods" is psychologically the way we face the fearful recesses of our collective menstrual mind, which believes we will perish if we don't perform certain rites of "tradition." By substituting metaforms, we successfully outrun not only our own habits but the "jackal" of our consciousness of what causes death and the legacy of traumatic blood that so closely accompanies human culture. Induced, or wound-caused, blood was itself a substitution—of men's blood transformed ritually into "menstrual" blood through parallel rites. This trickster principle of craft, this "craftiness," is one of the most creative in the human bag of menstrual *logos,* one we need more than ever.

Finally, we come to the sixth principle, crossing. (6) *Crossing* marks the great shifts of power between women's *r'tu* and men's parallel rites. Crossing takes advantage of the fact that the genders have different relationships to the central menstrual entrainment and therefore can trade leadership back and forth—like a shuttle on a loom. Because archaeology is unearthing the feminine past, origin story is crossing from males-only to a balanced, inclusive view that reintegrates the feminine and promises to incorporate the stories of everyone on earth.

The phrase "bread and roses" is from the early twentieth-century labor movement, in which women participated. I understand their demand for "bread and roses" to mean that sustenance—though fundamental and often hard to get—isn't enough for the harsh reality of life in the modern world. "Roses" are needed as well as "bread," enough income for some beauty and grace, some leisure and art, some vitality and fun, and for *cosmetikos*—that is hardly too much to expect in exchange for one's

275

labor. To these two I have added "blood," meaning recognition of female origin stories. The three vital elements are linked by the connective *and*, our contribution to the *logos* of science and religion.

The Way and the Way Back

The male tradition has "the way" to sally forth in a straight line, and women (led to great extent by feminists) have successfully followed men out of the strangling subjective matrix of the past. But men's undeviating path has also led us away from old truths and over a cliff, without "the way back." It is the women's tradition that holds the memory of the way back. The image of the arrow has dominated science and politics, but an arrow's path is only one direction. The "ascent of man" cannot be the whole story, for it omits the lessons of descent, of humility and renewal, and appreciation of the body's wisdom, nature's cycles, and the restrictions and celebrations of *r'tu*.

We need all the tools of humankind: arrow *and* loom, hierarchy *and* consensus, competition *and* cooperation, tenderness *and* ferocity, leisure *and* discipline. Men and women are not in deadly opposition. They are dancing the steps that give us human culture, that allow us to abstract "concepts" from our metaforms— nonsexual unions of the gender-minds. I believe the emergence of Gay movements in the twentieth century also signals a crossing, especially with the connection of lesbianism to female centrality and "flow."

The necroforms that hold in place racial, sexual, and other caste systems should be considered social and psychological pathologies that our scientists, linguists, poets, theologians, artists, historians, and healers can and should unravel as rapidly as possible. We need to substitute living metaforms for these destructive emblems. We need imagery and language, rites and emotional expressions that can "switch" our minds and return us to a sense of the ties between us. We are all here in the forms our ancestors revered because that was what kept their world together: long-necked swans, gap-toothed cows, black-skinned trees, knobby-faced rocks, round-faced suns, willowy-limbed snakes, blue-eyed skies, pale-cheeked moons, obsidian-eyed stones, hook-nosed hawks, broad-lipped ducks, red-haired carrots. We have all been shaped by our ancestral ideas, but now have new tools with which to see ourselves whole.

Although it may be "better to light a single candle than to curse the darkness," I say it is better still to uncurse the dark. We must learn the world whole. Light is evil as well as good; dark is good as well as evil. Semen, in the age of AIDS, can no longer be seen as "clean" and life-giving—penises have to be veiled in rubber now. Sunlight is dangerous, as are the toxic byproducts of materialist factories and the insecticides used to make perfect food. And the light of nuclear fission has eclipsed the old power of menstrual blood to destroy the world.

According to astronomers and physicists, light constitutes only about 7 percent of the cosmos, and the center of the sun is dark. "Light" can be said to exist only in the context of that greater dark. The All-god cannot possibly be only "light," then, for the cosmic mind operates largely in what is for us, with our dependence on our organs of sight, darkness. If deity is the known cosmos, it lives mostly in "the shade."

The seminal explosion of male-led technology of the last few centuries is being absorbed by women now. Men need to be excellent and fearless teachers; women need to know that men do not bring the final Word, the way they once brought home fire or a wild dog. We all must construct a new set of metaforms—forceful *r'tu* that performs some of the same functions as war but eliminates its sacrifice of humans and earth. Nuclear force, chemical waste, and acid rain can be brought under control if we remember how we've solved problems in the past, and that we've been given some marvelous new looms to weave new Words.

It is impossible for me not to believe that menstruation, entering a state of newly washed hygiene, will quickly entrain again with a different set of elements—those needed to neutralize the forces set

277

in motion by male seclusion and male-only origin story. Women, having learned what the male story offers, will become again teachers with a new set of "Female Instructing Principles." We will again find Snake, for menstruation is our most enduring covenant.

In the Gaia theory of biologists Lynn Margulis and James Lovelock, the self-regulating ecosystem has created an atmospheric shroud, as though the earth has veiled itself to regulate the life-shortening force of the sun. In a sense we, all organic life, are the earth's measuring forms. We are the cultural paraphernalia of "her" external mind and help to weave the veil that protects us all. Perhaps if we learn again the entrainments of fellow creatures and planetary bodies we will understand their Word, reconnect with them, and begin to see how we fit into the pattern. We must discipline intuition with objective scientific principles, so we can trust it and use it effectively in a new *dia logos*.

We materialist humans seem to be moving in a great procession, toward what destination, what new marriage, we do not know. Our Word is migrating once again. Having gone from skin to skirt, and then from skirt to script, it is now written on screens as dancing light with sound and color. But that light, like any other, can only exist in a context of interaction with dark; and in the microcosm, the pixels that build the characters and forms on the screen are honeycomb weavings of light *and* dark. The numerical system that stores the microchip information is a yes/no system.

The world created through digital video-computers—offers a potentially hopeful vision. As a network is set in place worldwide, we may soon work at home or some new version of home, where parents can be with their children, neighborhoods can develop again, where we can "materialize" reality in experiences of written light, without overprocessing the natural world, or so much parading in our fire-driven chairs. The new Word demands also a new basis of economy—what is it we have to trade from screen to screen? Is this a chance for different terms for the "washing" effect of money? For several hundred years in the West, money has been endowed with the seminal power to wash. It is "saved," held back

278

in "banks," as also blood is stored in blood "banks," and as earlier, water was seen as stored in river "banks." In banks, money took on a reproductive role and was given the ability to "increase and multiply" through such forms as interest and profit. Will money now be gauged in units of energy measured as computer time or microchip bytes as it was once gauged in units of gold, or salt, or red feathers? Why can't we even out the disparity between people with centralizing *r'tu* but no goods and the people who have goods but no centralizing *r'tu*? How can the earth be an economic partner who benefits from our endeavors?

Young people have always been catalysts of change, and sometimes eras that seem most difficult, when we are at the bottom of our Descent, are most valuable in the formulation of new *r'tu*. We need young Word brokers to help establish new systems of value and exchange. Meanwhile, the satellites catapulted from earth's surface by the Cold War have become an "eye of life." We have been given a view of our blue planet from off its surface. We can see it whole, measure our impact on it, and see its new patterns. The question is whether we can also learn to see from the point of view of the earth, of matter, and of all living beings.

The Great Wash of Shame

To hasten into consciousness the renewed menstrual mind, we might want to work with our residues of shame, which are completely related to menstrual knowledge. Shame is consciousness of ability to do evil, and it is a fundamental human quality. Shame is also acknowledgment of something unfinished, raw, and is therefore the doorway to creativity and finding solutions. Shame accompanied some great discoveries—of the harm of incestuous mating, of the power to transmit disease, of the power of semen in conception, of the reality of individual death, of the ability of human cultures to live without blood sacrifice.

Deep shames attach to being female, and they don't diminish when we drive our shiny cars out into the world chasing our arts

279

and sciences, learning and contributing to the new ways that men command them. We feel shame when we can't live up to all that is expected of us in family obligations, in the world, and in our own psychological and sexual persons. I have developed a women's shame ritual—based in a rite devised by my partner, Kris Brandenburger—that acknowledges the power of shame and frees our creativity and joy.

In a small group, two or three women set a date for the rite at least two weeks in advance. Each spends time thinking about her own shames, making a short list of them. She dresses for the rite in ragged, dirty, ill-fitting, or otherwise shameful clothes. At the appointed time, the women gather and sit facing each other, taking one long turn at a time telling their shames. Some women may want to cover their heads with a cloth while speaking, or to use other simple additions from their menarchal tradition. While the "menstruant" is speaking, the companion(s) listen, careful not to solve, interrupt, or negate the shame—letting it be what it is. Then others take turns with their own lists.

When all have spoken, the women go to a bath place—a large household shower or public hot tub or sauna, or a pond or lake— any body of water where they can take turns washing each other from head to foot, including the hair, and with special attention to the hands, feet, and face. Feelings of shame may accompany this portion as well, so silence may be enjoined.

After the bathing, the women dress in some of their best clothes, fix their hair, helping each other and admiring the clothes if they feel like it. Finally, they go out to dinner or to a special meal they prepare together, and enjoy themselves.

For a larger group of women who don't know each other very well, a group may begin with general discussions of some menstrual history and metaformic ideas, telling of individual experiences of menarche or childbirth, and of shame. The larger group breaks into units of four, six, or eight. Two women sit facing each other on the floor or ground, while the rest stand around them, facing each other in lines with their arms extended and fingers locked together, forming a hut shape in which the two seated ones are enclosed. Leave the east side open, and if there are as many as six "walls," the last pair can close in the west side. The walls can listen or not, as they choose.

After each "menstruant" has finished speaking her shame, the companion washes her face and hands with a clean cloth dipped in clean water. In my experience guiding women in this rite, the washing was a profound experience, and participants often wanted to take a long time with it.

When every pair has taken a turn as menstruant and companion, when everyone has told her shames, the group rearrange or change clothing, comb their hair, sit comfortably, and share some metaformic food—red fruits, dark breads, wine or beer or cola drunk with a straw—as reminders of where our lives originated and that we are woven together by our metaforms.

I imagine my next shame rite. In humility, I sit facing my companion sister Ereshkigal, surrounded by towering walls of the living female hut. "My father bought me a case of cosmetics when I was thirteen," I begin, "and I scorned it." Now I close my eyes to imagine my two parents, back in their garrulous mid-fifties, suspending their daily battle to sit so eagerly side by side in their living room, giving me the fragment of the oldest human tradition. They watch my face so closely—I feel again my grief and shock, and theirs.

And I reach again, taking the box, knowing this time I will use it in my own way. I embrace them each in turn for everything they gave me, and as everything that brought me here and connects me to the past. I will go out into the world of men to learn what is there. But I will also stay connected to women every chance I get, until we figure out what this little box will do for the world, once we open it.

Notes

1. How Menstruation Created the World

1. Briffault, *The Mothers*, vol. 2, p. 404.
2. See Jane C. Goodale, *Tiwi Wives*, and Margaret Mead, *Growing Up in New Guinea*.
3. See Grahn, "From Sacred Blood to the Curse and Beyond," in Spretnak, *The Politics of Women's Spirituality*, pp. 265–79.
4. In the Dakota language, the connection between "sacred" and "menstruation" is conveyed by the word *wakan*. See Briffault, *The Mothers*, vol. 2, p. 412. Shuttle and Redgrove in *The Wise Wound* also discuss this.
5. Dudley, "She Who Bleeds Yet Does Not Die," p. 112.
6. Knight, *Blood Relations*, pp. 246–49. Knight lists twenty-five nonhuman primates.
7. Thompson, *Tales of North American Indians*, p. 19.
8. Waters, *Book of the Hopi*, p. 1.
9. Euripides, Fragment Six of the *Melanippe*. This Greek text from a lost play by Euripides dates from the fifth century B.C. In Doria and Lenowitz, *Origins*, p. 168.
10. Hesiod, *Theogony*, quoted in Weigle, *Creation and Procreation*, p. 3.
11. Mountford, *Aboriginal Paintings from Australia*, p. 6.
12. Rawlinson, *Assyrian and Babylonian Literature*, p. 282. For a more recent translation, see Pritchard, *Ancient Near Eastern Texts*, pp. 60–72.
13. Durdin-Robertson, *The Goddesses of Chaldaea, Syria, and Egypt*, pp. 1–6.
14. Walker, *The Woman's Encyclopedia of Myths and Secrets*, pp. 998–99.
15. Genesis 1, King James Version (KJV), originally published as *The Good Leader Bible*.
16. Knight, "Menstrual Synchrony and the Australian Rainbow Snake," in Buckley and Gottlieb, *Blood Magic*, pp. 232–55.
17. See Hart, *Drumming at the Edge of Magic*, p. 121.
18. See the early study by Martha K. McClintock, "Menstrual Synchrony and

Suppression," *Nature* 229, no. 5282 (January 1971). McClintock's work is mentioned in Weideger, *Menstruation and Menopause,* pp. 34–35, and in Knight, *Blood Relations,* p. 213. Shuttle and Redgrove discuss several scientific experiments on light and "biological clocks" and suggest that the ritual of "drawing down the moon" of European wisewomen may relate to light and menstrual synchrony. They also cite research showing temperature synchrony of men to their female mates and among Gay male lovers. See *The Wise Wound,* pp. 162ff., 326–27.

19. Frazer, *The Golden Bough* (1929), vol. 2, p. 599.
20. Howey, *The Cat in the Mysteries of Religion and Magic,* p. 80. Howey continues, "Various derivations of the word Sabbath have been suggested, but perhaps none is quite convincing. In Hebrew the grammatical inflexions show that it is a feminine form, properly *shabbat-t* for *shabbāt-t.* The root carries no implication of resting in the sense of enjoying repose, but in transitive forms means to 'sever,' to 'terminate,' and intransitively means to 'desist, 'to come to an end.' It cannot be translated 'the day of rest,' but the grammatical form of *shabbath* suggests a transitive sense— 'the divider'—and would seem to denote that the Sabbath divides the month, or, in the case of the witches' quarterly festival, the year."
21. After appearance of Apsu and Tiamat, "Their waters commingling as a single body;/No reed hut had been matted, no marsh land had appeared" (Pritchard, *Ancient Near Eastern Texts,* p. 61). The Sumerian word for hut, *giparu,* applies to both a primitive woven dwelling and a "cult hut." In Sumerian moon temples, the *giparu* was the special temple precinct of the moon goddess, Ningal—so the "cult hut" was menstrual, as well as sacred, in its nature.
22. Frazer, *The Golden Bough* (1930), vol. 1, pp. 35–36.
23. Ebihara, "Khmer Women in Cambodia: A Happy Balance", in Carolyn Matthiasson, *Many Sisters.*
24. Frazer, *New Golden Bough,* p. 668.
25. Ibid., p. 669.
26. Beckwith, *Hawaiian Mythology,* p. 512.

2. Light Moved on the Water

1. *Oxford English Dictionary.* Perhaps Lucifer, god of All-light, fell from his high post after the solar religions deposed him as an obsolete idea.
2. Knappert, *The Acquarian Guide to African Mythology,* pp. 161–63.
3. Ibid., p. 165.
4. Wolkstein, and Kramer, *Inanna, Queen of Heaven and Earth,* p. ix.
5. Dundes, *The Flood Myth,* p. 163.
6. Goodale, *Tiwi Wives,* pp. 47–50.
7. People gave diverse reasons for these practices, citing the harm the menstruant could bring but also fear that she could be harmed: "Among the Parivarams of Madura, when a girl attains to puberty she is kept for six-

teen days in a hut . . . and when her sequestration is over the hut is burnt down and the pots she used are broken into very small pieces, because they think that if rain-water gathered in any of them, the girl would be childless" (Frazer, *New Golden Bough*, p. 669).

8. Briffault, *The Mothers*, vol. 2, p. 412. Briffault refers to Numbers 19:9 ff. and Leviticus 12:2. Numbers describes the sacrifice of a red calf and the proper method of sprinkling its blood and purifying one's hands and clothing afterward.

9. Denise L. Lawrence, "Menstrual Politics: Women and Pigs in Rural Portugal," Buckley and Gottlieb, *Blood Magic*, p. 267.

10. Ross, *Folklore of the Scottish Highlands*, pp. 75–77; Frazer, *The Golden Bough* (1930), vol. 1, p. 97.

11. Dundes, *The Flood Myth*, p. 164.

12. Ibid.

13. Guss, *The Language of the Birds*, pp. 60–70.

14. Frazer, *New Golden Bough*, p. 667. Frazer notes further: "Now it is remarkable that the foregoing two rules—not to touch the ground and not to see the sun—are observed either separately or conjointly by girls at puberty in many parts of the world."

15. Ibid., p. 668.

16. Ibid.

17. Mead, *Growing Up in New Guinea*, p. 112.

18. Frazer, *The Golden Bough* (1929), vol. 2, p. 598.

19. Frazer, *New Golden Bough*, pp. 667–68.

20. Heizer, *Handbook of North American Indians*, vol. 8, p. 565.

21. Frazer, *New Golden Bough*, p. 220 (emphasis added).

3. Crossing the Great Abyss

1. This creation story was related to me by Ilse Kornreich, an Argentinian poet, who said it came from indigenous people.

2. Frazer, *New Golden Bough*, p. 62.

3. Paula Weideger discusses this, *Menstruation and Menopause*, pp. 115–17, as does Chris Knight, *Blood Relations*, p. 428. See also Shuttle and Redgrove, *The Wise Wound*, p. 66. See also my article, "From Sacred Blood to the Curse and Beyond," in Spretnak, *The Politics of Women's Spirituality*.

4. Griaule, *Conversations with Ogotemmêli*, pp. 22–23. The Dogon equate the clitoris with the termite mound. They justify the operation with the argument that the clitoris is a "masculine" organ and if it is not excised it will grow long and prevent intercourse. In *Possessing the Secret of Joy*, Alice Walker describes the continuing impact of this crippling operation upon girls and women and suggests that it spreads AIDS, performed as it is with unsterilized, crude cutting instruments, including tin cans.

5. Schultz, *Hombu*, p. 29. Knight, *Blood Relations*, pp. 404–5, reports

that Yurok men's sweat lodges, which menstruants also had, were explicitly identified as the male equivalent of menstrual huts, and that men slashed their legs to bleed while they sweated.

6. Heizer, *Handbook of North American Indians*, vol. 8, p. 271.
7. Frazer, *New Golden Bough*, p. 224.
8. Ibid., p. 214.
9. Heizer, *Handbook of North American Indians*, vol. 8, pp. 240–41.
10. Begay, *Kinaaldá*, p. 97ff.
11. Judith Gleason, workshop on an African women's coming of age ceremony, at the Jung Institute, San Francisco, 1991. She stated that the ceremony occurs years after menarche and is not specified as menstrual.
12. See Heizer, *Handbook of North American Indians*, vol. 8, p. 328, for one of a number of examples.
13. See Walker, *The Woman's Encyclopedia of Myths and Secrets.* Scots-Canadian author Anne Cameron relates that the Scottish word *mon* referred to women until recently, and it originally referred only to women, men being called *wer* (personal communication).
14. See Aswynn, *Leaves of Yggdrasil:* "The term *men* in old Germanic languages, as for example in Anglo-Saxon, denoted not just the male section of the folk. The words for man and woman were 'weapmen' and 'weavemen' respectively; clearly the former means men with weapons, and the latter translated literally as 'men who weave,' i.e., women" (p. 89).

4. Wilderness Metaform

1. Frazer, *New Golden Bough*, p. 668.
2. Ibid.
3. See Briffault, *The Mothers*, vol. 2, p. 385; and Frazer, *New Golden Bough*, p. 668.
4. Briffault, *The Mothers*, vol. 2, pp. 418–19.
5. Knight, *Blood Relations*, p. 245. His theory is based in synchrony and sexuality, not the attraction of wild dogs to menstrual blood, however. "The earliest hominids . . . arose and for several million years evolved in the Rift Valley and along the shores of the Afar Gulf. Assuming that females were already tending to synchronize for sexual-political reasons . . . the ovarian cycles of closely associated females in this setting could hardly have escaped selection pressures to mesh in with the movements of the moon and any tidal rhythms, however slight."
6. Guss, *The Language of the Birds*, p. 70. This is related in a myth from the Guyana highlands of southern Venezuela, "They're not really dogs . . . but . . . packs of jaguars."
7. Knappert, *The Acquarian Guide to African Mythology*, p. 168.
8. Heizer, *Handbook of North American Indians*, vol. 8, p. 423.
9. Griaule, *Conversations with Ogotemmêli*, pp. 20–21.
10. Heizer, *Handbook of North American Indians*, vol. 8, p. 567.

11. This hypothesis is put forth convincingly by Chris Knight throughout *Blood Relations*.
12. See Walker, *The Woman's Encyclopedia of Myths and Secrets*, s.v. "Snake."
13. Mountford, *Aboriginal Paintings from Australia*, p. 12 (emphasis added). Mountford continues: "The Wandjina paintings feature beings that are eighteen feet in length with white, mouthless faces, surrounded by two horseshoe-shaped bows with radiant lines."
14. A drawing of this is in Vicki Noble's *Shakti Woman*.
15. Beckwith, *Hawaiian Mythology*, p. 289. Haumea also has a daughter named "Rosy Light in the Sky" (pp. 278–79), who can be seen as a metaformic creation of light from menstrual consciousness. Haumea has several forms and names, including "The Place of Blood" (p. 379).
16. Knappert, *The Acquarian Guide to African Mythology*, p. 221.
17. The Tantric tradition describes "Kundalini snake," inner body energy imagined as coils of a serpent at the base of the spine.
18. Knight, *Blood Relations*, p. 455. Knight describes a range of meanings for Rainbow Snake that includes "the mother of us all," creativity, power, and a time in the distant past.
19. Carnochan and Adamson, *Empire of the Snakes*, p. 111. Carnochan and Adamson described the thorns as an inch long, "strong as steel and sharp as a surgeon's needle." The rite took place in the bachelor hut, which only one old woman, "Snake-Mother," might enter; she brought the initiates food in a bowl. Being men the authors were not allowed near the women's Snake society rites.
20. Knappert, *The Acquarian Guide to African Mythology*, pp. 220–21, 235; Walker, *The Woman's Encyclopedia of Myths and Secrets*, s.v. "Coatlicue."
21. Robinson, *The Nag Hammadi Library*, p. 155. "The Hypostasis of the Archons."
22. In southern Ohio the "Serpent Mound," an earthen sculpture one-quarter mile long, attracts many tourists every year. The formation, which stands twenty feet wide and five feet high, is believed to have been built by the Hopewell people, who are no longer recognized as a separate tribe. It is an excellent example of a serpent form well on its way to becoming a dragon. The long body twists in seven lunar curves, and a spiral tail shows its connection to earth energy. Its head is flanked by two round shapes representing protruding eyes while the huge mouth is open like a vagina, in the act of enveloping or expelling a large egg shape. According to a knowledgeable Hopi man, the large triangle shape that lies beyond the egg is a "light catcher." He interpreted the egg-shaped mound as a village whose placement near the snake's mouth indicates that the people are under its protection. He said further that the size of the snake's body means it is the longest snake the people know, and that his name is Tokch'i, Guardian of the East. See Waters, *The Book of the Hopi*, p. 49.

287

23. Vollmer, *Five Colours of the Universe,* p. 18ff. Among other powers, the dragon regulated water, floods, and irrigation.
24. Rawlinson, *Assyrian and Babylonian Literature,* pp. 283–84.
25. The angel Michael fights the dragon in the Book of Revelation, but there the beast is male. "And behold a great red dragon, having seven heads and ten horns, and seven crowns upon his heads. And his tail drew the third part of the stars of heaven, and did cast them to the earth: and the dragon stood before the woman which was ready to be delivered, for to devour her child as soon as it was born" (Revelation 12:1–4 [KJV]).
26. In several seclusion rites branches were piled over the menstruant, or were placed at the opening of her hut, or she wore them around her waist or head.
27. Schultz, *Hombu,* p. 22.
28. Thompson, *Tales of the North American Indians,* p. 128.
29. "In the Tuhoe tribe of Maoris' the power of making women fruitful is ascribed to trees. These trees are associated with the navel-strings of definite mythical ancestors, as indeed the navel-strings of all children used to be hung upon them down to quite recent times" (Frazer, *New Golden Bough,* p. 115).

5. How Menstruation Fashioned the Human Body

1. Griaule, *Conversations with Ogotommêli,* p. 82. In describing women's beauty, Ogotommêli said that "to be naked is to be without speech."
2. Briffault, *The Mothers,* vol. 2, pp. 414–15.
3. Knight, in Buckley and Gottlieb, *Blood Magic,* p. 237.
4. Reed, *Woman's Evolution,* p. 98. See also Briffault, *The Mothers,* vol. 2, pp. 412–17: "Since woman's blood was taboo, daubing with blood became the mark or insignia of the tabooed condition. In the course of time red ocher came to serve as a substitute for blood."
5. Briffault, *The Mothers,* vol. 2, pp. 414–15.
6. Frazer, *New Golden Bough,* p. 668.
7. Douglas and Slinger, *Sexual Secrets,* pp. 241 and 352.
8. Briffault, *The Mothers,* vol. 2, pp. 390–96.
9. Reed, *Woman's Evolution,* pp. 135, 36.
10. Briffault, *The Mothers,* vol. 2, p. 397.
11. Frazer, *The Golden Bough* (1929), vol. 2, p. 600.
12. Daniëls, *Folk Jewelry of the World,* p. 32.
13. Fisher, *Africa Adorned,* p. 137. The Dogon balance of gender and the body is in Griaule, *Conversations with Ogotommêli.*
14. Daniëls, *Folk Jewelry of the World,* p. 84.
15. Heizer, *Handbook of North American Indians,* vol. 8, p. 540.
16. Ibid.
17. Handy and Pukui, *The Polynesian Family System in Ka-'u Hawaii,* pp. 10–11.

18. Sproul, *Primal Myths,* p. 334. In the male origin story cited by Sproul, the god Lowa sent two men to tattoo everything in the world, and this is how each kind of animal got its characteristic markings.
19. Heizer, *Handbook of North American Indians.* vol. 8, p. 688. Rock painting was explicitly included in menarchal rites of the Luiseño (p. 556).
20. Briffault, *The Mothers,* vol. 2, pp. 162—63. Briffault says the young Tuareg women protested vehemently, to no avail.
21. Ibid.
22. Ibid.

6. Cosmetikos and Women's Paraphernalia

1. Heizer, *Handbook of North American Indians,* vol. 8, p. 173, has an example.
2. Frazer, *The Golden Bough* (1930), vol. 1, p. 53.
3. See Pritchard, *Ancient Near Eastern Texts,* p. 37.
4. Douglas and Slinger, *Sexual Secrets,* p. 243: "Recent pharmacological research suggests that camphor stimulates the respiration, heart and cerebral cortex, and has a powerful effect on activating memory. Furthermore, scientific tests show that special preparations of camphor can increase clairvoyance."
5. Ibid., p. 242.
6. Grieve, *A Modern Herbal,* s.v. "Deadly Nightshade."
7. Frazer, *The Golden Bough* (1929), vol. 2, pp. 596—97.
8. Ibid., p. 597.
9. Gilbert, *Treasures of Tutankhamun,* p. 141.
10. Griaule, *Conversations with Ogotemmêli,* pp. 119—20.
11. Frazer, *The Golden Bough* (1930), vol. 1, p. 52.
12. Ibid., pp. 44—45. The cedar is a red-wooded tree, held sacred by many tribes.
13. Ibid., p. 20.
14. Ibid., pp. 47—48.
15. Ibid., p. 52.
16. See ibid., pp. 41, 48—49; also Heizer, *Handbook of North American Indians,* vol. 8, p. 327: "The Wintu menstruant was not supposed to leave her hut except at night. If she had to go out in the day, she covered her head with a basket or a hide." Frazer, *The Golden Bough* (1929) vol. 2, p. 600: "Amongst the Tlingit (Thlinkeet) or Kolosh Indians of Alaska, when a girl showed signs of womanhood she used to be confined to a little hut or cage. . . . She had to wear a sort of hat with long flaps, that her gaze might not pollute the sky; for . . . her look would destroy the luck of a hunter, fisher or gambler, turn things to stone, and do other mischief."
17. Briffault, *The Mothers,* vol. 2, p. 382.
18. Frazer, *The Golden Bough* (1930), vol. 1, p. 46, 49.
19. Linda Cassius, personal communication, 1992.

20. Griaule, *Conversations with Ogotemmêli*, pp. 19–21. In response to see-
    ing the earth's nakedness, the Nummo made a plant fiber skirt with ten
    long plaits in front and ten behind (ten for the fingers). The sinuous plaits
    were watery and flowing—and red. According to Ogotommêli, "the pur-
    pose of this garment was not merely modesty. It manifested on earth the
    first act of ordering the universe." And when the jackal again attempted
    to mate with the earth, he grabbed her skirt and got menstrual blood on
    it, and stained the earth as well.
21. Ibid., pp. 169–70. First the fibers were stolen, when "a woman got hold
    of them, put them on, spread terror all around her, and reigned as a
    queen, thanks to this striking adornment which no one had ever seen
    before." And then the men stole the fibers from the queen, and put them
    on in rites that excluded all but a few women.
22. Ibid., pp. 79–80. The ancestral warp of the woman's teeth separated the
    threads into eighty strands, representing the eighty Dogon ancestors—so
    all their history is carried in her face. Men also file their teeth, and only
    men do the weaving now, though women still spin.
23. Turkish women wore blue turquoise stones on their foreheads to ward off
    the "Evil Eye"; these were called "buts," which seems a possible early
    source of the word "button." (*Webster's* speculates goat's horn as source.)
24. Frazer has examples of women in childbirth eating with long sticks (*New
    Golden Bough*, p. 213). In one tribe, the menstruant was fed with a crab
    claw (*The Golden Bough* [1930], vol. 1, p. 37).
25. Ibid.
26. Frazer, *The Golden Bough* (1930), vol. 1, p. 42.
27. Frazer, *New Golden Bough*, p. 212.
28. Ibid., p. 596; "With the Awa-nkonde, a tribe at the northern end of Lake
    Nyassa, it is a rule that after her first menstruation a girl must be kept
    apart, with a few companions of her own sex, in a darkened house. The
    floor is covered with dry banana leaves." See also Schultz, *Hombu*, p. 24,
    for a description of the Tucuna tribe of the Amazon region.
29. Frazer, *The Golden Bough* (1929), vol. 2, p. 597.
30. Actually, she was only pretending to menstruate, as her father was search-
    ing her tent for some clay female images (teraphim) that she had stolen
    from him and hidden in the "camel's furniture"—a leather seat about two
    feet high. When he entered she said she could not rise, "for the custom of
    women is upon me. And he searched, but found not the images" (Genesis
    31:35 [KJV]).

7. Ceremony: Let's Cook!

1. Briffault, *The Mothers*, vol. 2, p. 389.
2. Ibid.
3. See Knight, *Blood Relations*, and Lévi-Strauss, *The Raw and the Cooked.*

4. Guss, ed., *The Language of the Birds*, pp. 5–9.
5. Frazer, *New Golden Bough*, p. 115.
6. Wolkstein and Kramer, *Inanna, Queen of Heaven and Earth*, p. 12.
7. See Evelyn Reed, *Woman's Evolution*, p. 116. Indigenous peoples, in Australia, for example, say that digging sticks "belong" to women. "Anthropologists also point to the fact that in the primarily horticultural economies of 'developing' tribes and nations, contrary to Western assumptions, the cultivation of the soil is to this day primarily in the hands of women" Eisler, *The Chalice and the Blade*, p. 69). United Nations reports on women farmers and the world economy, and mythology with its many associations of the female with plants and agricultural rites, all confirm the probable female origins of cultivation.
8. Grieve, *A Modern Herbal*, s.v. "Garlic."
9. On potatoes used as dyes, see Sauer, *Seeds, Spades, Hearths, and Herds*, p. 129. Sauer's general theory is that ceremonial purpose was at least as great a motive as desire for foodstuffs in the development of cultivation by women: In South America, "they colored food and painted themselves with the fruit of the Bixa, whence, perhaps, the origin of the name red Indians" (p. 42). "Southeast Asia included the spice lands of early commerce—and the emphasis on the coloring of food, person, and clothing, especially yellow or red (as by turmeric), with ceremonial significance attached thereto as life-giving, from birth through marriage to funerary offering" (p. 27).
10. Francia, *Dragontime*, p. 36.
11. Goodale, *Tiwi Wives*, p. 195.
12. Grieve, *A Modern Herbal*, pp. 161–66.
13. Ross, *Folklore of the Scottish Highlands*, pp. 147–50.
14. Meador, *Uncursing the Dark*, pp. 92–103.
15. Sauer, *Seeds, Spades, Hearths, and Herds*, pp. 48, 128–29.
16. Among some peoples, the idea of giving boys a menstrual, or visionary, state of mind was extended to include males at any time of life. A particular drug is planted, tended, harvested, and prepared exclusively by women among the Kogi people, said to be the last intact precolumbian agricultural tribe. But the drug, in white powder form, is eaten only by the men, who keep the powder with them at all times, in gourd containers they describe as "wombs." The powder induces a meditative state, teaching the men to concentrate on the religious principles of their people, to remind them to keep the old taboos and to remember the old ways in the face of encroaching modern society (see Ereira, *The Elder Brothers*, pp. 88, 92).
17. See Sauer, *Seeds, Spades, Hearths, and Herds*, p. 142. Also Katz and Maytag, "Brewing an Ancient Beer," p. 24.
18. Walker, *The Woman's Encyclopedia of Myths and Secrets*, p. 637.
19. Thanks to Anchor Steam Brewing company for sending this information, and the instructive poem, which they got from archaeologists when they

decided to repeat the recipe of Ninkasi in a beer of their own: Ninkasi beer. See Katz and Maytag, "Brewing an Ancient Beer."

20. "Medieval churchmen insisted that the communion wine drunk by witches was menstrual blood, and they may have been right. The famous wizard Thomas Rhymer joined a witch cult under the tutelage of the Fairy Queen, who told him she had 'a bottle of claret wine . . . here in my lap,' and invited him to lay his head in her lap" (Walker, *The Woman's Encyclopedia of Myths and Secrets,* p. 637). But the claret would have been drunk as a metaform for menstrual blood, just as Christian communion wine is a metaform for the blood of Jesus.

21. In a compound matrix of menstrual logic, "the same elixir of immortality received the name of *amrita* in Persia. Sometimes it was called the milk of a mother Goddess, sometimes fermented drink, sometimes sacred blood. Always it was associated with the moon. 'Dew and rain becoming vegetable sap, sap becoming the milk of the cow, and the milk then becoming converted into blood:—Amrita, water, sap, milk, and blood represent but differing states of the one elixir. The vessel or cup of this immortal fluid is the moon'" (Walker, *The Woman's Encyclopedia of Myths and Secrets,* p. 637).

22. Knappert, *The Acquarian Guide to African Mythology,* pp. 168–69.

23. This account is from Griaule, *Conversations with Ogotemmêli,* p. 150.

24. Gomme, *The Traditional Games of England, Scotland, and Ireland,* pp. 74–76. Also Jayakar, *The Earth Mother,* p. 60, explicitly states the rural Indian belief that an "essence" of sacrificial power passes from human sacrificial blood to blood of horses, goats, oxen, and sheep and is then found by digging in the earth, in rice and barley. Also, corn-grinding is part of menarchal seclusion rites among the Hopi (Ortiz, *Handbook of North American Indians,* vol. 9, p. 599). Thus at least the following grains have been related to menstrual *r'tu* or mythology as the "earth's blood": rice, barley, millet, emmer wheat, corn, and *fonio.*

25. Walker, *The Woman's Encyclopedia of Myths and Secrets,* p. 638.

26. Knight, *Blood Relations,* p. 414.

27. Ibid., p. 255. Along the southern California coast, Ipai and Tipai people "roasted" girls at menarche on beds of steaming leaves for a week. See Heizer, *Handbook of North American Indians,* vol. 8, p. 603.

28. Frazer, *The Golden Bough* (1930), vol. 1, p. 57.

29. Denise L. Lawrence, "Menstrual Politics: Women and Pigs in Rural Portugal," in Buckley and Gottlieb, *Blood Magic.*

30. Ibid., p. 124.

31. Ibid., p. 125.

32. Wolkstein and Kramer, *Inanna, Queen of Heaven and Earth,* p. 4.

33. Wooley, *Ur of the Chaldees,* p. 116.

34. Heizer, *Handbook of North American Indians,* vol. 8. Acorn cakes were often dyed red; the Miwok mixed red clay with acorn meal (p. 416); the

name of the Pomo means "at red earth hole" and includes the name for a hematite used to stain acorn meal red (p. 277).
35. Begay, *Kinaaldá*, p. 99ff.

8. Parallel Menstruations

1. Briffault, *The Mothers*, vol. 2, p. 366: "Premature births and all issues of blood are treated as regards tabu in the same manner as full-time births, and the reference to the cause of the tabu is always to the lochia and not to the child."
2. Heizer, *Handbook of North American Indians*, vol. 8, p. 422.
3. Linderman, *Pretty Shield*, pp. 128–29. Also Heizer, *Handbook of North American Indians*. vol. 8, p. 422. According to Heizer, Wappo women scored their flesh with their nails and with flint; the Wappo also had a special office of "grave robber" who dressed as a coyote and made coyote sounds (p. 268).
4. Translation of "The Descent of Inanna to the Underworld" by Betty DeShong Meador, in *Uncursing the Dark*, pp. 19–31, 46, 70–91.
5. Gimbutas, *The Language of the Goddess*. p. 158.
6. See Heizer, *Handbook of North American Indians*, vol. 8: Kitanemuk (p. 566); mourners were washed and given money and new clothes (p. 556); Luiseño ritually washed mourners' clothing (p. 556); Costanoan destroyed the deceased's hut (p. 491). See also traditions of the Tubatulabal (p. 440); Karok (p. 186); Foothill Yukuts (p. 480); Hupa (p. 173); Chimariko (p. 209).
7. Goodale, *Tiwi Wives*, pp. 47, 50–51.
8. Heizer, *Handbook of North American Indians*, vol. 8: Athapascan (p. 197); Wintu (p. 329); Yokuts (p. 455); Gabrielino (p. 545).
9. Frazer, *The Golden Bough* (1966), p. 106.
10. See Grahn, *Another Mother Tongue*.
11. Heizer, *Handbook of North American Indians*, vol. 8, has a number of examples.
12. Ahern, "The Power and Pollution of Chinese Women," in Wolf and Witke, *Women in Chinese Society*, p. 213.
13. Heizer, *Handbook of North American Indians*, vol. 8, p. 346: In the Nomlaki tribe it was said that "'pain' might be introduced into the body because of some breach of conduct (for example, 'fooling with a menstruating woman')."
14. Begay, *Kinaaldá*, pp. 63–65, 79, 85–87, 95, 105. She runs five times during the three-day ceremony, always toward the east.
15. Fisher, *Africa Adorned*, p. 116.
16. Bowles, *Autobiography of Jane Bowles*, p. 254.
17. Fischman, "Hard Evidence," *Discover Magazine*, pp. 44–51, on findings of Lewis Binford from a site in southwestern France.

18. Frazer, *The Golden Bough* (1966), part 2, pp. 198–99.
19. *Macmillan Dictionary of Historical Slang*, p. 723: "Prick," first recorded in 1592, was English slang for penis in the era before gunpowder, when spears, arrows, and other penile objects were primary methods of drawing blood.
20. The geographer Eduard Hahn proposed that the motive behind the domestication of horned animals was not economic but sacrificial, for use in religions connected to the moon. He suggested that milking and castrating were fertility rituals and that the horns of the animals selected for herding signified the lunar crescents. Since his controversial proposal others (Joseph Campbell, William Erwin Thompson, Carl Sauer) have also drawn the conclusion that the crescent horns of certain animals drew the attention of human hunters and led to domestication. To integrate this idea with mine, all but the most recent animal domestication—of horses and camels—appears to be intricately connected to the roots of religion through menstrual rite.
21. See Sauer, *Seeds, Spades, Hearths, and Herds*, pp. 30–31; and Campbell, *The Masks of God*, vol. 1, pp. 444–49.
22. Sauer, *Seeds, Spades, Hearths, and Herds*, pp. 89–90. Of twelve major large animals that have been kept by humans—pig, cattle, Zebu, water buffalo, goat, sheep, elephant, reindeer, yak, camels (two kinds, Bactrian and dromedary), horse, and ass—eight are horned or tusked. The horned were generally the earliest kept; the horse and camel were domesticated relatively recently as was the reindeer.

9. Sex, Matrimony, and Trickster Wolf

1. See Knight, *Blood Relations*, for an alternative, though in many ways overlapping, theory of menstrual seclusion as a female sex strike to acquire meat from hunters.
2. Walker, *The Woman's Encyclopedia of Myths and Secrets*, p. 556.
3. Wells, *A Herstory of Prostitution in Western Europe*, p. 41.
4. This version of the tale is from *The Complete Fairy Tales of the Brothers Grimm*, pp. 101–5.
5. Grieve, *A Modern Herbal*, s.v. "Oak."
6. Ibid., s.v. "Hawthorne."
7. Tatar, *Off with Their Heads*, p. 37.
8. Griaule, *Conversations with Ogotemmêli*, p. 156. The Dogon believe that the prepuce and clitoris are female and male parts, respectively, and must be removed so each sex is solely itself (and then can be "twinned" by marriage). These operations are also payments of "blood debts" (and sacrifice, especially of women) to the earth, and thus reflect menstrual reasoning applied to definitions of gender.
9. Goodale, *Tiwi Wives*, pp. 47–51.
10. In some Jewish weddings, both the bride and groom are carried about in

chairs. For a tribal parallel, see Mead, *Growing Up in New Guinea,* pp. 107–16. After several days of seclusion inside her mother's house, the young woman's family engaged in a series of feasts and giving of presents that involved the whole village. Her father threw coconuts into the sea, and distributed round balls of sago to other households. Her paternal grandmother fed her special foods, chased her through the house, and carried her down the household ladder on her back.

11. Tüzün, *Historical Costumes of Turkish Women,* pp. 63–64, 75–85.
12. Frazer, *The Golden Bough* (1930), vol. 1, pp. 48, 49, 50. Gleason, *Oyá,* p. 132.
13. Betty Bao Lord, *Spring Moon* (New York: Harper and Row, 1981).

10. Number, Orientation, and the Shapes of Light

1. Marshack, *The Roots of Civilization,* chap. 9.
2. Walker, *The Woman's Encyclopedia of Myths and Secrets,* pp. 645–46.
3. Marshack, *The Roots of Civilization,* chap. 10.
4. Ibid., chap. 13.
5. Heizer, *Handbook of North American Indians,* vol. 8, has examples.
6. Rossiya Fajardo, personal communication, 1992.
7. Gimbutas, *The Language of the Goddess,* chap. 11.
8. Ibid., chap 1, p. 12. See also Griaule, *Conversations with Ogotemmêli,* p. 81: Dogon women wear the "female number" incised in their foreheads in four parallel cuts, which are kept moist with oil because they are meta-formic of the vulva, and responsive to the Spirit of Water.
9. In Dogon culture, the marriage bed must have directional alignment. When they consummate their union, the married couple must lie on their sides facing each other on a bed that signifies "earth": the wife must face east, with her left hand resting on her husband's hip; he must lie facing west, with his right hand resting on her hip. See Griaule, *Conversations with Ogotemmêli,* p. 140.
10. See, for example, Terrell, *Indian Women of the Western Morning,* p. 141: "The more serious part of the ceremony took place inside a special tipi made for the girl. She danced continually, except for occasional rest pe-riods, until midnight, to the singing of a shaman and the shaking of his deer's foot rattle. On the fourth night, the dancing of the girl continued until dawn. When morning came the shaman painted the girl's face red, then made a dry 'painting' of the sun on his palm with pollen and other pigments, pressed this on the girl's head, and finally painted her arms and legs white. All the guests filed past, the shaman marked them in turn with some pigments. The girl raced to the east."
11. Walker, *The Woman's Encyclopedia of Myths and Secrets,* p. 673.
12. Howey, *The Cat in the Mysteries of Religion and Magic,* p. 68.
13. Knight, "Menstrual Synchrony and the Australian Rainbow Snake," in Buckley and Gottlieb, *Blood Magic,* p. 235. Initially they threw a string

loop (of synchroneity) around honey, the reddish liquid probably a meta-form of trees' (or bees') menstrual blood.

14. Ibid., p. 234; also Mountford, *Aboriginal Paintings from Australia,* p. 6.

15. Frazer, *The Golden Bough* (1929), vol. 1, pp. 79–80. This people also used a cup and ball game to bring the sun back more quickly in the spring. See in addition, Frazer, *The Golden Bough* (1966), p. 377: Everyone in the village of the Kiwai of Papua New Guinea played cat's cradles to pro-mote growth of the yam plants, and strings used to tie the yams were generally treated with "the usual medicine, fluid from the women's vulvae."

16. Kline, *Mathematical Thought from Ancient to Modern Times,* p. 11, and Hogben, *Mathematics for the Millions,* p. 215.

17. Tompkins, *Secrets of the Great Pyramid,* p. 194.

11. The Making of the Goddess

1. Frazer, *The Golden Bough* (1929), vol. 2, p. 597.

2. Frazer, *New Golden Bough,* p. 190.

3. Ereira, *The Elder Brothers,* p. 124ff. It is when the Mamas are most in seclusion that they are most in contact with the mind of the earth, *aluna.* In the hierarchy of sun priests, the most extremely secluded—living far more in the spirit world than in the material world—spend their lives on the tops of mountains, coming in contact only with other Mamas. They are oracles, then, perhaps similar in function to Greek Sibyls and priest-esses—the Pythia—at Dodona and Delphi, or to Celtic Druid priests, who were also kept in seclusion for years.

4. Frazer, *New Golden Bough,* p. 190. According to Frazer the capitol of the native king of Fernando Po (Bioko) was at the bottom of an extinct volcano, where the king lived with a priesthood of forty women. He could not use tobacco, rum, or salt. He was not allowed to see the sea even at a distance, and lived out his life with shackles on his legs in the dim light of his hut so he could not accidentally wander out and view it.

5. Ibid., pp. 190–91.

6. Frazer, *The Golden Bough* (1929), vol. 2, pp. 593–94.

7. Briffault, *The Mothers,* vol. 2, p. 373. Frazer, *The Golden Bough* (1929), vol. 2, p. 593: "Within his palace the king of Persia walked on carpets on which no one else might tread; outside of it he was never seen on foot but only in a chariot or on horseback." Perhaps the carrying of menstruants, brides, and royalty is a major reason for use of camels and horses (as well as carriages) being developed. According to the Oxford English Dictio-nary a light one-horse carriage was formerly called a "chair."

8. Frazer, *The Golden Bough* (1929), vol. 2, p. 594.

9. Griaule, *Conversations with Ogotemmêli,* p. 119.

10. Frazer, *The Golden Bough* (1929), vol. 2, p. 594.

11. Frazer, *New Golden Bough,* pp. 283–84, description of Cassange rite.

12. Graves, *The White Goddess*, p. 52.
13. Wolkstein and Kramer, *Inanna, Queen of Heaven and Earth*, p. 99.
14. Gimbutas, *The Goddesses and Gods of Old Europe*, pp. 72, 80.
15. The figure (from a site at Chatal Huyuk, c. 6000 B.C.E.) has been depicted many times, for instance in Gimbutas, *The Language of the Goddess*, p. 107.
16. *Oxford English Dictionary*, s.v. "Chair."
17. Paula Gunn Allen on the significance of how bangs are cut among Hopi maidens (personal communication, 1982).
18. Frazer, *New Golden Bough*, p. 117.
19. Kerényi, *Zeus and Hera*, pp. 143–44.
20. See Gimbutas, *The Language of the Goddess*, p. 70, for illustrations of the "snake goddesses."
21. Sauer, *Seeds, Spades, Hearths, and Herds*, p. 32.
22. Knappert, *The Acquarian Guide to African Myth*, p. 166.
23. Robert Graves, cited in Weigle, *Creation and Procreation*, p. 252.
24. Leviticus 15 : 28, 29 (KJV).
25. Fisher, *Africa Adorned*, p. 55.
26. She is especially well-depicted in Gadon, *The Once and Future Goddess*, plate 31; the color plate displays her red color.
27. Knight, *Blood Relations*, p. 364, see map. See also Marshack, *The Roots of Civilization*, and Gimbutas *Goddesses and Gods of Old Europe*. Knight also sees "seclusion" connoted in the bowed heads and hidden faces (p. 372). A photo of pale, weak menstruants emerging with heads bowed is in Schultz, *Hombu*, plate 62.
28. Weigle, *Creation and Procreation*, p. 33.
29. Tam Tro Graphics, 154 Garfield Place, no. 5, Brooklyn, N.Y. 11215.
30. Douglas and Slinger, *Sexual Secrets*, p. 354.
31. Ibid.
32. The Greeks grouped goddesses in threes, as they also divided their thirty-day month into three sections. See Kerényi, *Zeus and Hera*, pp. 121–23.
33. Ibid., pp. 114, 158–67.
34. Ibid., pp. 145–47, 97–98. I have greatly simplified Kerényi's account.

12. Menstrual Logic in the Visible World

1. Cohodas, "The Symbolism and Ritual Function of the Middle Classic Ball Game in Mesoamerica," p. 99 (emphasis added).
2. Ibid., p. 109.
3. Walker, *The Woman's Encyclopedia of Myths and Secrets*, p. 803.
4. Krupp, *Echoes of the Ancient Skies*, p. 84.
5. Ibid., pp. 84–88.
6. Frayne, "Notes on the Sacred Marriage Rite," pp. 5–22.
7. This is a composite description. The New Year's epic was read at Babylon. The preparations for the marriage of the *en*-priestess are from Frayne,

"Notes on the Sacred Marriage Rite," pp. 5–22. The Hymns to Inanna in Wolkstein and Kramer's *Inanna, Queen of Heaven and Earth,* pp. 93–110, are full of information about the processsions and offerings to Venus as morning and evening star.

8. See Grahn, *Another Mother Tongue,* chap. 4, on Halloween customs retained in Gay culture.
9. Meador, *Uncursing the Dark,* pp. 92–103.
10. Marglin, *Wives of the God King,* p. 234.
11. Ibid., p. 235.
12. Ibid.
13. Ibid., pp. 101–2: "On that day the Bathing festival (*Snāna Purnimā*) takes place, which inaugurates the car festival . . . which also corresponds with the breaking of the monsoon." See also pp. 234–35: "The songs which are sung by the women at that time are called Raja-swing songs. . . . The women perform a dance called Catki, which is considered the heart of the play during this festival. The men are not supposed to see this dance. The dance consists of the reenactment of a wedding, one girl dressing as a groom and one as a bride. All the women join in and the excitement reaches high peaks."
14. Ibid. The festivals are far more complex than I have suggested, and the role of the king and his *devadesis* priestesses (sacred harlots) is to bring about the rains through carefully timed sexual and dance ritual. Ceremonial presentation of food offerings and the separation of polluted from clean elements are adhered to meticulously by all the temple staff.
15. Walker, *The Woman's Encyclopedia of Myths and Secrets,* p. 139–40.

13. Narratives: Descent Myths and the Great Flood

1. New methods of dating stone archaeological evidence—thermoluminescence, electron spin resolution, uranium series dating—are pushing the dates of human development much farther into the past. Some archaeologists (Alison Brooks, John Yellen, Henry Schwarcz) suggest that complex culture existed in Africa as long as 100,000 years ago (Shreeve, "The Dating Game," pp. 76–83). Hélène and Georges Valladas—archaeologists of the French Atomic Energy Commission—have found Neanderthal (c. 60,000 B.C.E.) and Cro Magnon (c. 92,000 B.C.E.) flints in the same small area in Israel, suggesting the two physically—but not culturally—different peoples coexisted. (Until recently it was firmly believed that Cro Magnon had descended from Neanderthal). Their physical differences included capacity for speech: according to Jeffrey Laitman, an anatomical anthropologist at Mount Sinai School of Medicine, the physical ability to produce fully articulate speech stems from skull changes in which the larynx dropped down into the throat, producing a sounding chamber. The skull base started bending 1.5 million years ago, but not in the line classified as Neanderthals. These early humans lived between 130,000 and

35,000 years ago, made flints, used fire and perhaps (from pollen evidence) put flowers in graves, but the shape of their skulls suggests they could not use speech as we understand it. This supports Ogotemmêli's account—that Word was first a red skirt, and not spoken language. See Fischman, "Hard Evidence," pp. 44–51.

2. Knight, *Blood Relations*, pp. 392, 401.
3. Ereira, *The Elder Brothers*, p. 115.
4. Gimbutas, *The Language of the Goddess*, p. 19.
5. Inanna's city of Uruk dates from the fourth millennium B.C.E., though the most important information about her dates from 3500, along with "evidence of the earliest urban civilization. . . . the first truly monumental temple architecture . . . and the first writing" (Wolkstein and Kramer, *Inanna, Queen of Heaven and Earth*, p. 174). Merlin Stone, says the earliest examples of writing found in Inanna's temple at Uruk were at 3200 B.C.E. (*When God Was a Woman*, p. 40). Elinor Gadon (*The Once and Future Goddess*, p. 133) dates Inanna in the first half of the third millennium B.C.E. Thorkild Jacobsen (*The Treasures of Darkness*, pp. 21–26) has Inanna on a list of fourth millennium deities. He emphasizes Dumuzi's part in the sacred marriage, but of course the tradition of the ceremony was primarily Inanna's.
6. Good translations of the Descent myth are in Wolkstein and Kramer, *Inanna, Queen of Heaven and Earth*, and Meador, *Uncursing the Dark*.
7. See Wolkstein and Kramer, *Inanna, Queen of Heaven and Earth*, pp. 52–89.
8. Meador, *Uncursing the Dark*. Her translation retains the silence taboo. Wolkstein and Kramer use "Quiet, Inanna."
9. The poem is translated in Wolkstein and Kramer, *Inanna, Queen of Heaven and Earth*, pp. 12–27.
10. Ibid., p. 21.
11. I am using Gardner and Maier's translation of *Gilgamesh;* and also Pritchard, in "The Epic of Gilgamesh," in *Ancient Near Eastern Texts*, pp. 72–99.
12. Pritchard, *Ancient Near Eastern Texts*, p. 93. John Gardner's translation of the myth, though it has wonderful language and dense notes, omits the reed hut. Gardner calls it a "reed wall," as though Ea went to a marsh near the Persian Gulf to a figurative "wall of reeds" growing between land and sea. The reed hut, however, is explicitly in the Akkadian version, and this makes more sense if the myth is seen as menstrual—and therefore mythoreligious and mental—as well as naturalistic.
13. Genesis 6:15, 16 (KJV). The ark isn't square but rectangular—300 cubits long, 50 cubits wide, 30 cubits high, with rooms inside—and is made of wood and pitch. The Genesis ark is, like Ea's, three stories, with a door and window in the side.
14. Genesis 9:11–13 (KJV). The list continues (vv. 14–17): "And it shall come to pass, when I bring a cloud over the earth, that the bow shall be

299

seen in the cloud: And I will remember my covenant, which is between me and you and every living creature of all flesh; and the waters shall no more become a flood to destroy all flesh. And the bow shall be in the cloud; and I will look upon it, that I may remember the everlasting covenant between God and every living creature of all flesh that is upon the earth. And God said unto Noah, This is the token of the covenant, which I have established between me and all flesh that is upon the earth."

15. Exodus 25 (KJV).
16. Sanskrit "measure," *sar,* is also hidden in biblical Sarah.
17. Leviticus 15:29, 30 (KJV).

14. Crafting the Earth's Menstruation: Materialism

1. Jayakar, *The Earth Mother,* pp. 30–31.
2. Walker, *The Woman's Encyclopedia of Myths and Secrets,* pp. 866–67.
3. Robinson, *The Nag Hammadi Library,* pp. 169–70.
4. Leviticus 15:24, 33 (KJV).
5. Myth related by a Yurok woman in 1902. See Buckley and Gottlieb, *Blood Magic,* p. 194.
6. See Walker, *The Woman's Encyclopedia of Myths and Secrets;* Thass-Theinemann, *Symbolic Behavior,* pp. 197–208; and Heizer, *Handbook of North American Indians,* vol. 8, p. 186.
7. Griaule, *Conversations with Ogotemmêli,* pp. 197–208.
8. Buckley and Gottlieb, *Blood Magic,* p. 192.
9. Griaule, *Conversations with Ogotemmêli,* p. 87.
10. Walker, *The Woman's Encyclopedia of Myths and Secrets,* p. 150.
11. Wolkstein and Kramer, *Inanna, Queen of Heaven and Earth,* p. 54.
12. Ereira, *The Elder Brothers,* pp. 93, 229. Also de Camp, *The Ancient Engineers,* p. 234: The goldsmiths of Sumer used techniques of electroplating, using a battery of copper and iron rods in a salt solution, so the gold particles adhered to the surface of any object dropped into the bath. Electroplating was not discovered again until many centuries later. The battery, too, was kept in clay jars, as though, like the Kogi they so much resembled, the Sumerians and other Mesopotamian peoples also considered gold to be the earth's menstrual blood.
13. Ereira, *The Elder Brothers,* p. 157.
14. Ibid.
15. Ibid., pp. 158–59.
16. Jayakar, *The Earth Mother,* pp. 60–61.
17. Wolkstein and Kramer, *Inanna, Queen of Heaven and Earth,* p. 37.
18. Katz and Maytag, "Brewing an Ancient Beer," p. 29.
19. Heizer, *Handbook of North American Indians,* vol. 8, p. 343.
20. Griaule, *Conversations with Ogotemmêli,* pp. 95–97. As Chris Knight pointed out, the men's sweathouse was modeled after the menstrual hut. All this suggests that the sacred women's seclusion hut, which in many

cultures needed to be rebuilt after each use, was the basic original structure of the human village. See *Blood Relations,* pp. 404–5.

21. Handy and Pukui, *The Polynesian Family System in Ka-'u Hawaii,* pp. 10–11.
22. Kerényi, *Zeus and Hera,* p. 157.
23. See Meador, *Uncursing the Dark,* p. 95, who cites W. Burkert, *Greek Religion* (Cambridge: Harvard University Press, 1985).
24. Perring and Perring, *Then and Now,* pp. 110–15. The Teotihuacan temple complex included, besides the Pyramid of the Moon, a Pyramid of the Sun, a temple dedicated to the feathered serpent god Quetzalcoatl, and the Jaguar Palace.
25. Krupp, *Echoes of the Ancient Skies,* pp. 298–99. The complexity of sacred measurements embodied in temple architecture is best exemplified by the Great Pyramid of Egypt. "It has been shown to be a theodolite, or instrument for the surveyor, of great precision and simplicity, virtually indestructible. It is still a compass so finely oriented that modern compasses are adjusted to it, not vice versa" (Tompkins, *Secrets of the Great Pyramid,* p. xiv).
26. Ibid., p. xiii.
27. Ibid., p. 189ff.
28. Ibid., pp. 5–6.
29. Ibid., pp. 15–19, 63.
30. Ibid., pp. 26, 28, 64.
31. Inanna's emblematic hut is flanked by two tall reed columns shaped in circles at the top—two trees topped by streaming full moons with the dark moon hut between.

15. Crossing the Abyss to Male Blood Power

1. The work of Marija Gimbutas, James Mellaart, Sir Leonard Wooley, and other archaeologists forms the basis of physical evidence. Some researchers argue that Neolithic awe of woman's ability to bear children, coupled with a belief in her innate kindness, resulted in the eventual deification of women's nurturing and "life-giving" capacities. This seems to me a simplification that sentimentalizes the feminine as tender and benevolent and the masculine as inherently violent and dominating. Such stereotypes reproduce the myths of romantic and warlike patriarchal cultures. In this view, the "Goddess Mother" represents only "life," and her associations with death, sacrifice, and murder are ignored. Riane Eisler's description of Neolithic culture is typical: "Symbolized by the feminine Chalice or source of life, the generative, nurturing, and creative powers of nature—not the powers to destroy—were . . . given highest value" (*The Chalice and the Blade,* p. 43). Eisler and many others have credited "the power to destroy" exclusively to men, to "the Blade."
2. Weideger, *Menstruation and Menopause,* p. 115.

3. Beckwith, *Hawaiian Mythology,* p. 530.
4. Knappert, *The Acquarian Guide to African Mythology,* pp. 161–62.
5. Griaule, *Conversations with Ogotemmêli,* p. 193.
6. Ibid., pp. 193–94. The ritual thieves of the Dogon nowadays steal sheep and poultry to commemorate the smith's daring theft of fire. Such thefts often require ritual payments. Perhaps a male ritual tradition also existed in older times around the stealing of young animals from the wild. I am reminded that a shepherd's "crook" is also a term for thief in English. That ritual stealing may be an extension of menstrual rite is suggested by the fact that horse stealing was a part of the carrot festival of my mother's ancestors in Scotland. See Ross, *The Folklore of the Scottish Highlands,* pp. 148–49.
7. Genesis 30–31 (KJV) relates a story of Jacob's "stealing" his father-in-law's herd by arranging the breeding to come out in his favor. He had been given any "speckled cattle" born to the herd, and he used selective breeding to make sure the young were speckled more often than not.
8. See Evans, *Witchcraft and the Gay Counterculture;* Sjöö, *The Great Cosmic Mother;* and Walker, *The Woman's Encyclopedia of Myths and Secrets.* Ancient Snake/Satan is still venerated, his rites kept intact by a small priesthood in the hills of Syria who say that the powers of darkness must be remembered. Satan lives in a cave, where they tend him in his serpent form. (This cult is not to be confused with underground Satanism in the United States, which reportedly practices violence, torture, and abuse of women and children.)
9. Robinson, *The Nag Hammadi Library,* p. 130.
10. Walker, *The Woman's Encyclopedia of Myths and Secrets,* p. 815. "India's Kali Ma was the same creating-and-destroying Goddess, with a special incarnation as Kel Mari the Pot Goddess. Since she made the first man out of clay, her people were Aryans, from *arya,* 'man of clay.' Kel Mari was related to Mari of Mesopotamia, or Mariamne, or Miriam, or Mary, whose name was connected with the deaths of both John the Baptist and Jesus. Her earth, which drank the blood of sacrificed men, might have been the same Aceldama that drank the blood of Judas."
11. Jayakar, *The Earth Mother,* p. 60. See also p. 39: "The carpenter ministrants . . . break the glass bangles on the goddesses' wrists, strip them naked, take the red powder off their brows, pull off their heads, hands, and legs, and put them into the baskets. Then, mourning the death of the divine ones, they carry the baskets to the goddesses' temple and lay them in the idol room for three days." In many other places, goddess statues had removable limbs and head.
12. Pickthall, *The Meaning of the Glorious Koran,* Surah 81:8–9: "And when the girl-child that was buried alive is asked/For what sin she was slain . . ."
13. Diamond, "The Arrow of Disease," p. 66: "Smallpox, flu, tuberculosis,

malaria, plague, measles, and cholera—are all infectious diseases that arose from diseases of animals."

14. Ibid., p. 73.
15. Marija Gimbutas, cited in Eisler, *The Chalice and the Blade,* p. 45.
16. Jayakar, *The Earth Mother,* pp. 37–40.
17. Robbins, *The Encyclopedia of Myths and Secrets,* s.v. "Sexism." See also Briffault, *The Mothers,* vol. 2, p. 387: In the nineteenth century, people of the Lake Tanganyika region of Africa believed that consumption was caused by a menstruant's kindling a fire.
18. Walker, *The Woman's Encyclopedia of Myths and Secrets,* p. 187. "In the 17th century A.D., Christian writers still insisted that old women were filled with magic power because their menstrual blood remained in their veins. This was the real reason why old women were constantly persecuted for witchcraft" (p. 641).
19. Robbins, *The Encyclopedia of Witchcraft and Demonology,* p. 193.
20. Yet as late as the 1800s it existed in Scotland. Old women called "gallas"—(hence "gals"?)—mourned professionally, an office recorded in ancient Sumerian myth as that of *gallaturra* or *gallas.* See Ross, *The Folklore of the Scottish Highlands,* p. 115, and Wolkstein and Kramer, *Inanna, Queen of Heaven and Earth,* p. 191.
21. Noble, *World without Women,* p. 163.
22. Sheldrake, *The Presence of the Past,* pp. 23–28, and chap. 2 generally.
23. Frazer has many examples of taboo associated with war games and male sacrifice. He believed such games as football were once sacrificial. Baseball also has metaformic elements. Originally, the game was English "rounders," played with four pegs as bases (Seymour, *Baseball: The Early Years,* pp. 4–6). The ball, white with red stitching, is lunar. After three strikes (dark moon) the player is "out" ("dead" in menstrual terms). If the player's stick (tree) lifts the ball in a long enough arc (full moon), it goes off the field and the player runs "home." When four (number of the earth) balls are pitched wide, the player walks the base path—perhaps in earlier times oriented toward the four directions. One player's turn may be "sacrificed" in an easy out for the good of the team. Chewing tobacco and beer are part of baseball's mystique.
24. MacCulloch, *The Religion of the Ancient Celts,* pp. 178–79.
25. Ross, *The Folklore of the Scottish Highlands,* p. 25.
26. Lorde, *Sister Outsider,* p. 112.

Bibliography

Ackerman, Diane. *The Natural History of the Senses*. New York: Random House, 1990.

Ahern, Emily, "The Power and Pollution of Chinese Women." In *Women in Chinese Society*, edited by Margery Wolf and Roxane Witke, p. 213. Palo Alto: Stanford University Press, 1975.

Alexander, Hartley Burr. *The World's Rim: Great Mysteries of the North American Indians*. Lincoln: University of Nebraska Press, 1953.

Aswynn, Freya. *Leaves of Yggdrasil*, St. Paul: Llewellyn Publications, 1990.

Beckmann, Petr. *A History of Pi*. New York: St. Martin's Press, 1971.

Beckwith, Martha. *Hawaiian Mythology*. Honolulu: University of Hawaii Press, 1982 (first published 1940).

Begay, Shirley M. *Kinaaldá: A Navajo Puberty Ceremony*. Rough Rock, Ariz.: Rough Rock Demonstration School, 1983.

Benson, Elizabeth P. *The Maya World*. New York: Thomas Y. Crowell Company, 1967.

Briffault, Robert. *The Mothers*, 3 vol. London: Macmillan Company, 1969 (first published 1929).

Buckley, Thomas, and Alma Gottlieb, eds. *Blood Magic: The Anthropology of Menstruation*, Berkeley: University of California Press, 1988.

Budge, E. A. Wallis. *Osiris and the Egyptian Resurrection*. New York: Dover Publications, 1973.

———. *The Egyptian Book of the Dead*. New York: Dover Publications, 1967.

Campbell, Joseph. *The Masks of God: Primitive Mythology*. New York: Viking Press, 1972.

Carnochan, F. G., and Hans Christian Adamson, *The Empire of the Snakes*. New York: Frederick A. Stokes Company, 1935.

Carson, Anne. "Putting Her in Her Place: Woman, Dirt, and Desire." In *Before Sexuality: The Construction of Erotic Experience in the Ancient Greek*

World, ed. David M. Halperin, John J. Winkler, and Froma I. Zeitlin. Princeton: Princeton University Press, 1990.

Cartwright, Frederick F. *Disease and History.* New York: Dorset Press, 1972.

Cohodas, Marvin. "The Symbolism and Ritual Function of the Middle Classic Ball Game in Mesoamerica." *American Indian Quarterly* 2, no. 2 (Summer 1975); 99–130.

Culpepper, Emily, "*Niddah:* Unclean or Sacred Sign?" Unpublished paper, 1973.

Daniëls, Ger, ed. *Folk Jewelry of the World.* New York: Rizzoli International Publications, 1989.

Day, Cyrus Lawrence. *Quipus and Witches' Knots.* Lawrence: University of Kansas Press, 1967.

De Camp, L. Sprague. *The Ancient Engineers.* New York: Dorset Press, 1990.

Diamond, Jared. "The Arrow of Disease." *Discover* 13, no. 10 (October 1992): 64–73.

Diop, Cheikh Anta. *The African Origin of Civilization.* New York: Lawrence Hill and Company, 1974.

Doria, Charles, and Harris Lenowitz, eds., *Origins: Creation Texts from the Ancient Mediterranean.* Garden City, N.Y.: Anchor Books, 1976.

Douglas, Nik, and Penny Slinger. *Sexual Secrets.* New York: Destiny Books, 1979.

Dudley, Rosemary J. "She Who Bleeds, Yet Does Not Die." *Heresies,* no. 5 (1978).

Dundes, Alan, ed. *The Flood Myth,* Berkeley: University of California Press, 1988.

Durdin-Robertson, Lawrence. *The Goddesses of Chaldaea, Syria, and Egypt.* Cesara Publications, Ireland.

Ebihara, May. "Khmer Women in Cambodia: A Happy Balance." In *Many Sisters,* edited by Carolyn Matthiasson. New York: Free Press/Collier Macmillan, 1974.

Eisler, Riane. *The Chalice and the Blade.* San Francisco: Harper and Row, 1988.

Ereira, Alan. *The Elder Brothers.* New York: Alfred A. Knopf, 1992.

Evans, Arthur. *Witchcraft and the Gay Counterculture.* Boston: Fag Rag Books, 1978.

Fierz-David, Linda. *Women's Dionysian Initiation.* Dallas: Spring Publications, 1988.

Fischman, Joshua. "Hard Evidence." *Discover* 13, no. 2 (February 1992).

Fisher, Angela. *Africa Adorned.* New York: Harry N. Abrams, 1984.

Francia, Luisa, *Dragontime.* Translated from the German by Sasha Daucus. Woodstock, N.Y.: Ash Tree Publishing, 1991.

Frayne, Douglas R. "Notes on the Sacred Marriage Rite." *Bibliotheca Orientalis* 42, no. 1/2 (January–March 1985).

Frazer, Sir James George, *The Golden Bough: A Study in Magic and Religion.* Part 2, *Taboo and the Perils of the Soul.* Part 4, *Adonis, Attis, Osiris,* vols.

1 and 2. Part 5, *Spirits of the Corn and of the Wild,* vol. 2. Part 6, *The Scapegoat.* Part 8, *Bibliography and General Index.* Aftermath: *A Supplement to The Golden Bough.* New York: St. Martin's Press, 1966.

———. *The New Golden Bough.* New York: Criterion Books, 1959.

———. *The Golden Bough: The Magic Art.* Vol. 1. London: Macmillan and Company, 1932.

———. *The Golden Bough: Balder the Beautiful.* 2 vols. London: Macmillan and Company, 1930.

———. *The Golden Bough.* 2 vols. New York: Book League of America, 1929.

———. *Folklore in the Old Testament.* Vol. 1 London: Macmillan and Company, 1919.

———. *The Golden Bough: The Dying God,* London: Macmillan and Company, 1911.

Gadon, Elinor W. *The Once and Future Goddess.* San Francisco: Harper and Row, 1989.

Gardner, John, and John Maier, trans. *Gilgamesh.* New York: Vintage Press, 1985.

Gilbert, Katharine Stoddert, ed. *The Treasures of Tutankhamun,* New York: The Metropolitan Museum of Art, 1976.

Gimbutas, Marija. *The Language of the Goddess.* San Francisco: Harper and Row, 1989.

———. *The Goddesses and Gods of Old Europe.* Berkeley: University of California Press, 1982.

Gleason, Judith. *Oya: In Praise of the Goddess.* Boston: Shambala Publications, 1987.

Golub, Sharon, ed. *Lifting the Curse of Menstruation.* New York: Harrington Park Press, 1985.

Gomme, Alice B. *The Traditional Games of England, Scotland, and Ireland.* London: Thames and Hudson, 1984.

Goodale, Jane C. *Tiwi Wives.* Seattle: University of Washington Press, 1971.

Grahn, Judy. *Another Mother Tongue: Gay Words, Gay Worlds* Boston: Beacon Press, 1984.

Graves, Robert. *The White Goddess.* New York: Farrar, Strauss, and Giroux, 1973.

Griaule, Marcel. *Conversations with Ogotemmêli.* London: International African Institute/Oxford University Press, 1965.

Grieve, Mrs. M. *A Modern Herbal: The Medicinal, Culinary, Cosmetic and Economic Properties, Cultivation and Folk-lore of Herbs, Grasses, Fungi, Shrubs and Trees with All Their Modern Scientific Uses.* 2 vols. New York: Dover Publications, 1971 (first published 1931).

Grimm, Jacob, and Wilhelm Grimm. *The Complete Fairy Tales of the Brothers Grimm.* Translated by Jack Zipes. New York: Bantam Books, 1987.

Gump, Richard. *Jade: Stone of Heaven.* Doubleday and Company. Garden City, N.Y.: 1962.

Günay, Umay. *Historical Costumes of Turkish Women.* Istanbul: Middle East Video Corporation, 1986.

Guss, David M. ed. *The Language of the Birds.* San Francisco: North Point Press, 1985.

Handy, C. S. Craighill, and Mary Kawena Pukui. *The Polynesian Family System in Ka-'u Hawaii.* Rutland and Tokyo: Charles E. Tuttle Company, 1972 (first published 1958).

Harding, M. Esther. *Woman's Mysteries.* New York: Harper Colophon Books, 1971.

Harris, Rivkah. "Inanna-Ishtar as Paradox and a Coincidence of Opposites." In *History of Religions.* Chicago: University of Chicago Press, 1991.

Harrison, Jane Ellen. *Epilegomena to the Study of Greek Religion, and Themis.* New Hyde Park, N.Y.: University Books, 1962.

Hart, Mickey. *Drumming at the Edge of Magic.* San Francisco: Harper and Row, 1990.

Hawkins, Gerald S. *Stonehenge Decoded.* Garden City, N.Y.: Dell Publishing, 1965.

Heizer, Robert F. *Handbook of North American Indians.* Vol 8, *California.* Washington, D.C.: Smithsonian Institution, 1978.

Highwater, Jamake. *Myth and Sexuality.* New York: Meridian, 1991.

Hindu Myths: A Sourcebook Translated from the Sanskrit. London: Penguin Books, 1975.

Hoare, F. R. *Eight Decisive Books of Antiquity.* New York: Dorset Press, 1991.

Hogben, Lancelot. *Mathematics for the Millions.* New York: W. W. Norton and Company, 1983.

Hooper, Alfred. *Makers of Mathematics.* New York: Random House, 1948.

Hopkins, E. Washburn. *Epic Mythology.* Delhi: Motilal Banarsidass, 1915.

Howey, M. Oldfield. *The Cat in the Mysteries of Religion and Magic.* Rutland, Vt.: Charles E. Tuttle Company, 1981.

Hubbard, Ruth. *The Politics of Women's Biology.* New Brunswick: Rutgers University Press, 1990.

Hubel, David H. *Eye, Brain, and Vision.* New York: Scientific American Library, 1988.

Jacobsen, Thorkild. *The Treasures of Darkness: A History of Mesopotamian Religion.* New Haven: Yale University Press, 1976.

James, E. O. *The Cult of the Mother Goddess.* London: Thames and Hudson, 1959.

Jayakar, Pupul. *The Earth Mother: Legends, Ritual Arts, and Goddesses of India.* San Francisco: Harper and Row, 1990.

Katz, Solomon H., and Fritz Maytag. "Brewing an Ancient Beer." *Archeology* 44, no. 4 (1991): 24.

Kerényi, C. *Zeus and Hera.* Princeton: Princeton University Press, 1975.

———. *Goddesses of Sun and Moon.* Dallas: Spring Press, 1979.

Kline, Morris. *Mathematical Thought from Ancient to Modern Times*. New York: Oxford University Press, 1972.

Knappert, Jan. *The Acquarian Guide to African Mythology*. Northhamptonshire, England, 1990.

Knight, Chris. *Blood Relations: Menstruation, and the Origins of Culture*. New Haven: Yale University Press, 1991.

———. "Menstrual Synchrony and the Australian Rainbow Snake." In *Blood Magic*, ed. Thomas Buckley and Alma Gottlieb. Berkeley: University of California Press, 1988.

Koltuv, Barbara Black. *The Book of Lilith*. York Beach, Maine: Nicholas-Hayes, 1987.

Kramer, Heinrich, and James Sprenger, *Malleus Maleficarum*. London: Arrow Books, 1971.

Krupp, E. C. *Echoes of the Ancient Skies*. New York: Harper and Row, 1983.

Lander, Louise. *Images of Bleeding*. New York: Orlando Press, 1988.

Laubin, Reginald, and Gladys Laubin. *The Indian Tipi*. New York: Ballantine Books, 1957.

Levy, Gertrude Rachel. *The Gate of Horn*. London: Faber and Faber, 1948.

Linderman, Frank B. *Pretty Shield*. Lincoln: University of Nebraska Press, 1972.

MacCulloch, J. A. *The Religion of the Ancient Celts*. London: Constable and Company, 1991.

McNeill, William H. *Plagues and Peoples*. New York: Anchor Books, 1977.

Maddux, Hilary C. *Menstruation*. New Canaan, Conn. Tobey Publishing Company, 1975.

Marglin, Frederique Apffel. *Wives of the God-King*. Oxford: Oxford University Press, 1985.

Marshack, Alexander. *The Roots of Civilization*. Mount Kisco, N.Y.: Moyer Bell, 1991.

Matthiasson, Carolyn, ed. *Many Sisters*. New York: Free Press/Collier Macmillan, 1974.

Mead, Margaret. *Growing Up in New Guinea*. New York: William Morrow/Mentor Books, 1953.

Meador, Betty DeShong. *Uncursing the Dark*. Wilmette, Ill.: Chiron Publications, 1992.

Mellaart, James. *Catal Huyuk*. New York: McGraw-Hill, 1967.

Meltzer, David, ed. *Birth: An Anthology of Ancient Texts, Songs, Prayers, and Stories*. San Francisco: North Point Press, 1981.

Mitchell, John. *Secrets of the Stones*. Rochester, Vt.: Inner Traditions International, 1989.

Moortgat, Anton. *The Art of Ancient Mesopotamia: The Classical Art of the Near East*. London: Phaidon Press, 1969.

Mountford, Charles P. *Aboriginal Paintings from Australia*. Milan: United Nations Educational, Scientific and Cultural Organization, 1964.

Noble, David F. *A World without Women: The Christian Clerical Culture of Western Science.* New York: Alfred A. Knopf, 1992.

Noble, Vicki, *Shakti Woman.* San Francisco: Harper and Row, 1991.

Nowak, Margaret, and Stephen Durrant. *A Tale of the Nisan Shamaness.* Seattle: University of Washington Press, 1977.

Opie, Iona, and Moira Tatem, eds. *A Dictionary of Superstitions.* Oxford: Oxford University Press, 1992.

Ortiz, Alfonso. *Handbook of North American Indians.* Vol. 9, *Southwest.* Washington, D.C.: Smithsonian Institution, 1979.

Partridge, Eric, ed. *The Macmillan Dictionary of Historical Slang.* New York: Macmillan Company, 1974.

Patai, Raphael. *The Hebrew Goddess.* KTAV Publishing House, 1967.

Perring, Stefania, and Dominic Perring. *Then and Now.* New York: Macmillan Company, 1991.

Pickthall, Marmaduke. *The Meaning of the Glorious Koran.* New York: Dorset Press, 1954.

Pritchard, James B., ed. *Ancient Near Eastern Texts Relating to the Old Testament.* Princeton: Princeton University Press, 1969.

Rawlinson, Sir Henry, trans. *Assyrian and Babylonian Literature.* New York: D. Appleton and Company, 1901.

Reed, Evelyn. *Woman's Evolution.* New York: Pathfinder Press, 1957.

Reifenstahl, Leni. *People of Kau.* New York: Harper and Row, 1976.

Reiter, Rayna R., ed. *Toward an Anthropology of Women,* New York: Monthly Review Press, 1975.

Robbins, Rossell Hope. *The Encyclopedia of Witchcraft and Demonology.* New York: Crown Publishers, 1959.

Robinson, James M., ed. *The Nag Hammadi Library.* New York: Harper and Row, 1977.

Roessel, Ruth. *Women in Navajo Society.* Rough Rock, Ariz.: Navajo Resource Center, 1981.

Roscoe, Will. *Living the Spirit: A Gay American Indian Anthology.* New York: St. Martin's Press, 1988.

Ross, Anne. *The Folklore of the Scottish Highlands.* London: B. T. Batsford, 1990, (first published 1976).

Sauer, Carl O. *Seeds, Spades, Hearths, and Herds.* Cambridge: MIT Press, 1972.

Schultz, Harald. *Hombu.* New York: Macmillan Company, 1962.

Seymour, Harold. *Baseball: The Early Years.* New York: Oxford University Press, 1960.

Sheldrake, Rupert. *The Presence of the Past: Morphic Resonance and the Habits of Nature.* New York: Vintage Books, 1989.

Shreeve, James. "The Dating Game." *Discover* 13, no. 9 (September 1992): 76–83.

Shuttle, Penelope, and Peter Redgrove. *The Wise Wound: The Myths, Realities, and Meanings of Menstruation.* New York: Bantam Books, 1990.

310

Sjöö, Monica, and Barbara Mor. *The Great Cosmic Mother*. San Francisco: Harper and Row, 1987.

Spretnak, Charlene, ed. *The Politics of Women's Spirituality*. Garden City, N.Y.: Anchor Press, 1982.

Sproul, Barbara, ed. *Primal Myths: Creation Myths around the World*. San Francisco: Harper and Row, 1991 (first published 1979).

Stone, Merlin. *When God Was a Woman*. Dial Press, New York, 1976.

Sturluson, Snorri. *The Prose Edda*. Berkeley: University of California Press, 1954.

Talent, Robert. *Mardi Gras*. Gretna, La.: Pelican Publishing Company, 1976.

Tatar, Maria, *Off with Their Heads!* Princeton: Princeton University Press, 1992.

———. *The Hard Facts of the Grimms' Fairy Tales*. Princeton: Princeton University Press, 1987.

Taylor, Dena. *Red Flower: Rethinking Menstruation*. Freedom, Calif.: Crossing Press, 1988.

Terrell, *Indian Women of the Western Morning*. New York: Dial Press.

Teubal, Savina J. *Sarah the Priestess*, Athens, Ohio: Swallow Press, 1984.

Thass-Thienemann, Theodore. *Symbolic Behavior*. New York: Washington Square Press, 1968.

Thompson, Stith, ed. *Tales of the North American Indians*. Bloomington: Indiana University Press, 1972.

Thompson, William Irwin, ed. *Gaia, a Way of Knowing: Implications of the New Biology*. Great Barrington, Mass.: Lindisfarne Press, 1987.

———. *The Time Falling Bodies Take to Light*. New York: St. Martin's Press, 1981.

Tompkins, Peter. *Secrets of the Great Pyramid*, Harper & Row, Publishers, New York, 1971.

Tüzun, Özcan. *Historical Costumes of Turkish Women*. Istanbul: Middle East Video Corporation, 1986.

Vollmer, John E. *Five Colours of the Universe: Symbolism in Clothes and Fabrics of the Ch'ing Dynasty*. Alberta: Edmonton Art Gallery, 1980.

———. *In the Presence of the Dragon Throne: Ch'ing Dynasty Costume (1644–1911) in the Royal Ontario Museum*. Toronto: Royal Ontario Museum, 1977.

Von Franz, Marie-Louise. *Creation Myths*. Zurich: Spring Publications, 1972.

Walker, Barbara G. *The Woman's Encyclopedia of Myths and Secrets*. San Francisco: Harper and Row, 1983.

Waters, Frank. *Book of the Hopi*. New York: Ballantine Books, 1963.

Weideger, Paula. *Menstruation and Menopause*. New York: Dell Publishing Company, 1977.

Weigle, Marta. *Creation and Procreation*. Philadelphia: University of Pennsylvania Press, 1989.

———. *Spiders and Spinsters*. Albuquerque: University of New Mexico Press, 1982.

311

Wells, Jess. *A Herstory of Prostitution in Western Europe*. Berkeley: Shameless Hussy Press, 1982.

Wheelwright, Joseph B. *The Reality of the Psyche*. New York: G. P. Putnam's Sons/C. G. Jung Foundation for Analytical Psychology, 1968.

Wolkstein, Diane, and Samuel Noah Kramer. *Inanna, Queen of Heaven and Earth*. New York: Harper and Row, 1983.

Woodward, Kenneth L. "Swing Low, Sweet Chariot." *Newsweek*, June 10, 1991.

Wooley, C. Leonard. *The Sumerians*. New York: W. W. Norton, 1965.

———. *Ur of the Chaldees*. Melbourne: Penguin Press, 1954 (first published 1929).

Wyman, Leland C. *Blessingway*. Tucson: University of Arizona Press, 1987.

Index

315